The Personality Diet

The Personality Diet

The Simple Solution to Getting Off the Diet Hamster Wheel and Finally Creating Lasting Results

Mike Millner

Published by Game Changer Press, LLC DBA Game Changer Publishing

ISBN: 9798636925439

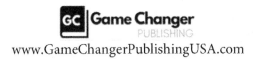

www.GameChangerPublishingUSA.com

Dedication

This book is dedicated to Pop-Pop. My hope is to impact at least a fraction of the amount of people you did throughout your life. I have felt your presence with me throughout this journey and could not have done this without you. Thank you for being my guiding light. The ripple effect you left on this world is still being felt today

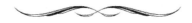

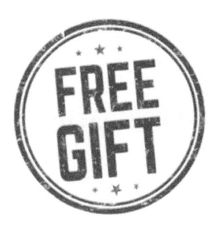

DOWNLOAD YOUR FREE GIFTS

Read This First

Just to say thanks for buying and reading my book, I would like to give you a free bonus gift that will add value and that you will appreciate, 100% FREE, no strings attached!

To Download Now, Visit:

http://www.personalitydietbook.com/MM/freegift

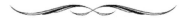

The Personality Diet

The Simple Solution to Getting Off the Diet Hamster
Wheel and Finally Creating Lasting Results

MIKE MILLNER

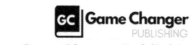
GC Game Changer
PUBLISHING
www.GameChangerPublishingUSA.com

Table of Contents

Foreword

THE TRUTH - As a coach, the only thing I can truly do is help my clients find the truth, tell the truth, and hope that they will lead their clients to the truth.

Enter Mike Millner.

I was first made aware of Mike on social media.

His name would pop up on some posts I made, and in return, I made sure to follow the posts he was making.

One thing was clear - he was extremely intelligent and extremely passionate.

But if I'm being honest, that didn't exactly differentiate him from many of the other coaches I had met.

Fortunately for Mike, it didn't stop there.

The first day I got to spend with him was in Chino Hills, California. If there was an award for the least number of words spoken in a classroom, he would've won that day. However, if there was another award for strongest presence in a room, he would've won that too.

Leaders don't always need to speak, they lead with their actions - and I knew that day that Mike was a LEADER.

What I also found out in the 10 hours that we spent together is that Mike operates at the highest levels of integrity and TRUTH.

At the conclusion of our day, Mike was presented with an opportunity to leave his current employer, start his own business, and make considerably more money almost immediately. For most, this is a no-brainer and a decision they don't think twice about - but not Mike.

Instead, he asked how we could actually take advantage of this opportunity while still continuing to help his current employer - going so far as to ask if there was a way we could give them a percentage of profits.

In well over a decade of networking with, and leading business owners, I can tell you that this was a FIRST (and currently, a last).

Why would he do this?

Simple - It was the right thing. But as I'm sure you are aware, knowing the right thing and doing the right thing are not always synonymous.

At this moment, I knew Mike was going to do amazing things in our industry. His commitments to success were not selfish - they were rooted in truly helping elevate everything and everyone around him.

He provides the TRUTH to his clients - ultimately setting them free.

He operates inside of TRUTH with other business owners - ultimately allowing him to become a leader and connector in a crowded industry.

And what follows in this book are principles based on TRUTH - finally giving you the tools and resources you need to create success.

In a world full of confusion, Mike is a bright light of clarity - and our industry is better because of him, his beliefs, and his passion to serve.

THANK YOU Mike, and thank you to everyone for your commitments to the TRUTH that this book will provide you.

Best of luck in your journey

Jason A. Phillips

"The Coach of Coaches"

CHAPTER 1

ARE YOU A SLAVE TO THE DIET INDUSTRY AND HAS THE DIET INDUSTRY FAILED YOU?

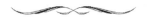

I'm not going to mention the name of this individual, because the who is not important. In fact, let's pretend that it's me. It was always a childhood dream of mine to be a professional athlete so at least I can play one in my own book. The statistics I'm about to share are very real. I'm simply implanting myself into the story. There I am, a major league baseball player with a massive salary. I signed a huge contract because of my ability to hit. Multi-millions being sent my way to be able to put the bat on the ball. Unfortunately, things didn't go as planned for me in this particular season of my career. I ended up posting a batting average of .168 in 522 plate appearances, which is the worst batting average in MLB history amongst qualified players. To put this in perspective, I was paid an 8 figure salary to succeed less than twice in every 10 at-bats that year. Can you imagine getting paid that much money to fail a little over 80% of the time? Well, that pales in comparison to the statistics of the diet industry. The worst batting average in a sport that has statistics dating back to the 1800s would be considered a massive success when it comes to dieting. Not only that, but the compensation for that historically poor performance is pennies when we look at the multi-billions spent on diets. We're talking about a $72 billion dollar industry that produces the following results: for every 10 people that embark on a diet journey, half of a person will succeed. I wonder which half? It's not a lack of funding and it's not a lack of access to information. It's a foundationally and fundamentally flawed system. So when you hear me say the words, are you a slave to the diet industry, I know that might sound extreme, but when you actually dig a little bit deeper and understand the manipulation that happens within the diet industry and the many millions of people that are affected by how dieting is done today, you understand that the word 'fits.' We're dealing with manipulation on a psychological and physiological level. One of the best ways to explain this is that a very successful weight loss company openly claims that the reason they're successful is because their clients leave them and then feel the need to come back. They brag about their clients not being able to maintain their weight loss as if it's a positive thing. However, if the goal is to lose weight and sustain it, then why would those clients feel the need to come back to this weight loss program? The answer is very simple. It's because they were unsuccessful. They put the weight back on, as do 95% of the people that try to diet. 95% will lose weight and gain it back. About one third to two thirds of the people will actually gain back more weight than they originally lost.

What that means is that the client felt like they were the failure. In other words, they didn't put the blame on the program they tried. They put the blame on themselves. They felt the need to go back to that program and it created a dependency on rules, restrictions, and the typical diet mentality. It's making you believe that you are the failure, whereas the reality is that the diet industry has failed you. It is a system that sets you up for failure. And the reason is that you're required to follow somebody else's rules.

Every single diet program out there is established in the same way. It's a set of rules or regulations that you have to follow and it doesn't factor in who you are as a person. It doesn't factor in any of the individual variables that make you unique. In other words, your lifestyle, your mindset, your current habits, your personality, what experiences are important to you in life, none of that is factored in. It's just very black and white. Here's our system, here are the rules you have to follow, and it's often a very restrictive type of way of living that is very difficult to become a lifestyle. As humans, when we're required to follow specific rules without factoring in our own individual variables, we are guaranteed to fail most of the time. We're dealing with a very well-funded, very smart, intelligent oppressor. I use that word because we need to break free from the way that things are currently done.

But there is hope. Liberation is right on the other side of understanding your own individual needs. We've seen examples of breaking free from oppression to create a better solution. It takes a movement. It takes an understanding that the current way isn't working and that we are not going to tolerate the current standards. You deserve better. We deserve better. We don't have to tolerate the way that things are currently done, we don't have to tolerate being manipulated in such a way that our psychological and physiological health is at risk. The statistics are clear that we are getting sicker and we are getting more obese year over year. Chronic illness is on a steady incline, obesity is on a steady incline and yet we continue to do things the same way and expect a different result.

I have some clients that I work with and some of their stories and my personal story also reiterate the fact that we need to do things differently. One of my clients, Danielle, shared her story with me about how she was in her 20s and was doing a very low carb plan, similar to the Atkins diet. Danielle said, "I lost around 80 pounds in six months and felt really happy and thought things were going well." Then she says everything physically fell apart. "It was unsustainable. I started gaining weight back super-fast plus interest, and it took years to get healthy again." She mentioned that her relationship with food, specifically carbs, was completely damaged. She was afraid to eat carbs because she associated them with weight gain. She had a poor relationship with her body at that point because she felt like a failure. It took her decades to get to the point where she felt better. Fortunately, we've worked together and she's been able to eat carbs and not have any guilt or shame associated with them and has lost weight in a healthy, sustainable way, but there is a lot of damage that needed to be undone. Looking at one of my other clients, Shantel, she said she had too many dieting horror stories to even count. She did her own version of a diet by only eating apples and rice because that's what she thought she needed to do. She thought she needed to be that restrictive in order to lose weight. She did an ultra-low-carb plan, which she said absolutely destroyed her and is still very vocal about the health impact it has and her doctors even suspect that it kicked her into hormonal disruption and early menopause. So, we're really talking about deep-rooted psychological and physiological damage. She even had a personal trainer, who recommended that she only eat twice per day and each meal would be three eggs, a half pack of bacon, one bell pepper and that was it.

She has now undone a lot of that damage through understanding her own personal needs. And I think that the point that's most important is that there is no such thing as a one-size-fits-all approach. There is no such thing as the best diet for everyone. And that is where the diet industry fails a lot of people, it's trying to make something that is multi-faceted, very personal, very individual and trying to create this one way of doing things and trying to fit everybody into the same box when we all have personal and individual needs. I actually learned this through my own journey. I was formerly 250 pounds and realized that I wanted to make a change because I didn't feel like myself. I was losing confidence. I had a lot of insecurities and I went on my weight loss journey shortly after college when I was 250 pounds and started doing things the way that the diet industry promotes. I started restricting calories, doing a lot of cardio, and I would get down below 200 which for me, was like this magic number that I wanted to achieve. Every time I got below 200, I would end up rebounding above 200 and I repeated this process for years. I'm talking like five years of yo-yo dieting, of gaining and losing and gaining and losing and every single time, I felt even more like a failure. It just reiterated the fact that I was not successful, that I couldn't do this, that maybe being fit and healthy just wasn't for me. Eventually, I started to understand that I shouldn't be following somebody else's rules. Eventually, I realized that I shouldn't be trying to do things the way that everybody else is doing them. Because again, when you look at the statistics, it's pretty clear that the way that we're being sold, the way that we're being told to diet is not going to work long term.

I started researching as much as I possibly could. The common denominator that I found, through all of my years of research and certifications and education, was that there was not going to be a one size fits all approach. I had to find my own way and look at who I am as a person, what's meaningful in my life, what does my lifestyle look like? What habits are serving me? Where is my mindset? Then establish a way of doing things that I could sustain for the rest of my life. It took me the better part of a decade to get there. I think a lot of people go through that process because it's so easy to fall into the quick-fix and the promises of fast results. The diet industry loves to pull on those emotional heartstrings. They love to draw you in with promises of quick weight loss and unbelievable results. It's human nature that we're typically impatient. We want results like yesterday and so we see these promises, we see these advertisements for losing weight fast and feeling better, and all a sudden we want to jump into the next best thing. But the problem is we fall into that same trap of playing by somebody else's rules. It wasn't until I started to create my own rules that the system of personality dieting came to be. It's basically an anti-diet approach to dieting where you can still achieve all of the goals that you have for yourself within your health and nutrition but it's going to factor in who you are as an individual, which allows for greater adherence, greater consistency. and greater sustainability. At the root of it all, those are going to be the key factors in determining long-term success. Do you actually enjoy what you're doing? Can you sustain this for the rest of your life? And are you able to adhere to that process almost effortlessly?

Now, there is work that needs to be done. There's a lot of things we can learn when we look at the five percenters. The people that have successfully lost weight, and kept it off for more than three years. They all employ some form of restraint, sacrifice, and self-control. However, they don't rely solely on those things. They view what they're doing truly as a lifestyle. The 5%, they also have a method to track progress. That can look differently depending on the individual, but they assess their results in some way. What gets tracked, gets changed. We have to pay attention to what's happening, so we know if we're moving in the right direction or not. It's important that you know from a mindset perspective, to truly view what you're doing as a lifelong solution. And that's something that the five percenters all have in common. They don't feel like they need to jump from diet to diet because they enjoy the process and what they're currently doing. One other thing that the five percenters have in common is that they maintain a training routine. As basic as that sounds, it's an important part of the process because your habits will dictate your results and so having a healthy habit in place, like some form of training, is very beneficial. Now, the interesting thing about this is that you'll see amongst the five percenters that some of them train more often than others. Some of them prefer weight training over cardio, some of them prefer cardio over weight training. The bottom line is that just having the habit in place of some form of training or exercise routine is a consistent variable when it comes to being successful with overall weight loss and living a healthier life.

The best way, in my opinion, to train for everyone is the way that you enjoy the most and that's a pretty simple thing. If you're miserable at the gym, you're not gonna do it for very long. If you are doing training and moving your body in a way that you love... Now, that's going to be very sustainable.

Another thing they have in common is structure. There's a Ben Franklin quote that says, "if you fail to plan you are planning to fail." So the five percenters have structure in their life and that can be something as simple as a morning routine or starting each day with a win. It could be having a glass of water in the morning, it could be going for a 10-minute walk, it could be doing some meditation or reading 10 pages of a book, etc. Something that starts your day in a structured fashion and having a plan throughout your day.

Another thing that I think is greatly overlooked, but we see is a common denominator for successful dieters, is the ability to delay gratification. This is super important when we're dealing with the diet industry because there's going to be a lot thrown at you that promises quick solutions. Successful dieters don't allow their short term feelings to get in the way of their long term goals. They may feel discouraged on a day where their weight fluctuates up, but they have the ability to not let that impact their actions and that is key. They understand the big picture. They can continue with their daily actions and habits that will eventually get them to where they want to be. That's super important from a mindset perspective because things are never going to be smooth sailing. In fact, chaos is more the norm than it's not. We know that life is always going to happen, which is why we have to keep things in perspective and understand what truly matters to us. Even something as small as delaying the short term satisfaction of the candy bowl at work, for the long term gain of achieving your goals of better health. It's just one simple example of the ability to delay gratification in the name of what you're trying to accomplish.

Successful dieters are generally turned off by fad dieting. They understand that the key to long term success is long term sustainability. So they don't do any form of extreme dieting or very restrictive protocols and that's something we can definitely learn and apply to ourselves.

Another thing that's often overlooked is social support. Successful dieters typically have some form of social support in place. Now, this can be tricky because, if you've ever been in a situation where you're with a group of friends, and they tell you what you should be doing, like, hey, it's okay, you can have a few drinks, you can eat this burger and fries, and they almost try to impact your behavior in a negative way. So it's important to choose carefully when you're looking at your social support system, even just something like one accountability partner or training partner, or being a part of a community where everybody's pursuing the same goal, that can make the process more fun, and more sustainable. Cultivating your environment to make it more prone to be successful, can really be an effective strategy. Sometimes tough decisions need to be made if you have a toxic person in your life, who is not supportive of your goals and you may need to have some difficult conversations. But it is very important.

The last thing I want to mention about the five percenters is that they have the ability to avoid the all or nothing mindset. This is something we see so commonly in dieters today. They're either all in or they're all out. That was my reality for years, which is why I talked about my yo-yo dieting, and that's where it all stemmed from. I felt like I needed to be absolutely perfect on every single diet program that I did. And the minute that I slipped up, it was just an epic failure. It was binge eating, it was stress eating, it was emotional eating, and then I would have to start back at square one. So we know that avoiding that all or nothing mindset, finding something that fits within who you are as a person, will help you find that balance and find that moderation without feeling like you need to be perfect.

Another way to help manage the all or nothing mindset is to practice gratitude along the way. As you're going through this process, you're going to have ups and downs but just being grateful for your ability to go through the process of trying to accomplish better health is a really effective strategy for avoiding that all or nothing thinking. Those are some of the similarities when we look at the five percenters who are successful in long term dieting, and I think at the root of it, it's just understanding that we all have individual needs, that we are all different people, and we shouldn't be approaching dieting as a one size fits all way of doing things. Your success cannot be found in somebody else's rules. What we need to do is lean into who you are as a person, your personality type, your mindset, your lifestyle, your current habits, your current goals and we look at all of those individual factors and then we can create your own way of doing things that will lead to your own success. That is what we've created with the personality diet. That's exactly what you're going to learn how to do.

CHAPTER 2

PERSONALITY DIETING

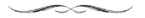

The whole concept of personality dieting began with my own journey and research. Once I understood and witnessed that each individual has their own set of unique needs, it became clear that traditional methods of dieting would continue to fail. The reason nothing has worked for you in the past is that you've been trying to play by somebody else's rules. When we look at the different methodologies and the various diets that are out there, they're all a different version of the same thing. There's going to be some form of control and manipulation that is placed upon you, regardless of which program you choose. It doesn't matter if it's time-restricted feeding, which would be a set eating window, for example, you can only eat from 12 pm to 8 pm. It doesn't matter if you're limiting certain types of foods like a very low-carb or no-carb plan. It doesn't matter if it's more of a food quality approach like you can only eat clean foods, for whatever that means as a definition. All of these different methodologies apply restriction to your intake in some way, shape or form. The issue with that is that we're not factoring in who you are as a person, which will help us accomplish the most important variable... sustainability.

Now, there is the possibility that you stumble upon a methodology that actually fits you perfectly, but the odds of that happening are very slim because we are all different. In the example of time-restricted feeding, if you're somebody who wakes up and you're very hungry in the morning, so you like to have breakfast to start your day. Plus, you've got a busy day at work and you want to have more energy to handle your day to day activities, then having to delay eating until noon or later is going to be a disaster for you. And that's just one lifestyle factor that we should look at when we're talking about what protocol will work best for you.

There are some people, based on how their schedule is set up, that it makes sense for them to skip breakfast, and maybe it even helps them feel better. Maybe it just fits within their lifestyle. However, the issue is when we try to create a way of doing things and apply it across the board to the masses. We know very specifically that that doesn't work. These methods are all just tools in a very large tool box and you would never pick the same tool to accomplish every job that needs to get done. You would look at the context and application of the situation and then choose the best tool for the job. In dieting circles, we see this constant search for the "one way" that will work best for everyone. Which is the same as saying that a hammer is always going to be the right tool for the job, regardless of whether you're trying to drive a nail into some wood or secure a screw? They're not factoring in critical context like who you are as an individual, what your current lifestyle looks like, what your habits are, and what you actually enjoy doing. That typically leads to diet hopping. I'm sure you can just think about your own personal experience. How many diets have you tried up to this point in your life? For me, it's probably upwards of 20 and that's a conservative estimation. I started on a very low calorie, low carb approach. Then I moved to more of a clean eating approach where I actually had a list of foods that I could and couldn't eat. Yes, I actually had a list of foods that were off-limits. Never mind the fact that from a physiological standpoint, it wasn't doing me any good. But think about the psychological damage that happens when you view foods as good versus bad. When you have this list of foods that you can't eat. Now all of a sudden, you only want to eat those foods that are off-limits. And that was my reality. The minute that I ate a food that was off-limits, I felt like I had to eat all of it because I knew that it was going to be taken away from me again. I call that last chance syndrome. Well, I better get this in while I can, because this is the last chance for me to eat this food before it's removed again.

This black and white thinking, this all or nothing mindset is typically what we go through and when we inevitably fail, we jump to the next diet. The next diet is just another protocol that outlines a whole other set of rules, and a whole other way of doing things that were established by somebody else. Now we're following a different system and the result is going to be the same. The statistics are super clear that if we just continue to jump from diet to diet, we're going to end up in the same place or even worse. What nobody talks about is how your personality actually impacts your ability

17

to stay consistent within a certain protocol. We know this to be true because there are certain people who do really well with certain strategies like time-restricted feeding. Certain people do really well with low-carb dieting. Certain people do really well with more of a paleo approach. The difference is that those people view it as a lifestyle. It's effortless to them because it fits within their personality type. So when we talk about personality dieting, it's really just a way of saying we're going to look at the characteristics and the traits that make you who you are as a person and we're going to align your nutrition and your fitness to accommodate those individual variables. At the end of the day, we're going to assess your personality, lifestyle, mindset, habits, goals, and personal preferences to pick the right tools for the job. It's going to look different for everybody but the process is much more effective and much more enjoyable. It's a simple shift from playing by somebody else's rules to creating your own rules that you actually want to be doing.

Most diets that you've tried in the past have required you to white knuckle your way through them. You have to rely on discipline and willpower and just buckle up and get it done. Which typically leads to feeling like a failure. Each time you fail a diet, you're reiterating in your mind that you are a failure and the confidence that you have to go into the next diet gets lower. Have you ever thought about trying a new program but you start to replay that same story in your mind? The story that you've failed before and this time won't be any different? That's the psychological damage caused by continuing down the path of traditional dieting. We have to break out of that mindset. It's not until we realize that we have to lean into who we are as individuals and find the way that allows for the greatest level of consistency within our own life, that we can truly break free from the way that diets are currently established.

Your personality will tell us a lot about consistency and how to frame that within your own life. It will tell us what you will adhere to and what will actually be the most enjoyable for you. When you see arguments about what diet is best, you won't even entertain those conversations because they won't apply to you. You'll understand it's an irrelevant argument. The question that you should be asking yourself is, is this approach best for me? Does this fit within my lifestyle? Does this account for the things that are meaningful in my life? In other words, can you still have a social life with your current protocol? Are you still able to do the things that are meaningful to you? Maybe it's travel, maybe it's date night, maybe it's getting pizza with the family, etc. Things that fulfill your health in another way outside of just physical health that are super important to the overall big picture. Does your current protocol allow for that? When we look at personality dieting, that is the root of it all. We want to account for who you are as a person and the things that you value to establish a protocol that is actually enjoyable and gets you the results that you want. The feeling should be effortless. It should feel like you're not actually dieting. It should feel like something you can do for the rest of your life. And when we're able to build in the framework of consistency to accommodate for things you love, like travel, dining out, going out with friends, you're not going to feel like you're failing your diet. Because you'll be living a life in total alignment.

That is the success that we've been able to create with thousands of personality diet based transformations. We assess each individual and learn who they are. Then we build in the consistency practices based on personality type which gives us better adherence, more sustainability, and more enjoyability, which is really an overlooked part of the process. This shouldn't be something that makes you miserable. I know that oftentimes we associate dieting with restriction but I'd like to reclaim the word dieting. The way that the diet industry uses the word dieting, we often think of restriction and deprivation and misery. Like it's something that we just have to do. Almost like it's a punishment for being human and wanting to look and feel better. The way that I think of dieting, is in terms of foods that nourish you, foods that allow you to thrive. It's eating in a way that allows you to be the best version of yourself. It's a protocol that allows you to enjoy your life and still achieve the results that you want. It's freedom. It's the opposite of restriction. It's breaking out of the handcuffs that the diet industry has placed on you and finding your own solution. It's never having to feel like you need to diet again. That is the way that we should be using the word diet because the technical definition is simply just the foods and drinks that we consume on a regular basis.

They use diet in terms of restriction. We use diet in terms of nourishment. They use diet to get you to be less. We use diet to get you to be more. They use diet as deprivation. We use diet as freedom. They use diet as an ideology. We use diet as a means for personal enhancement. They use diet to narrowly focus on calories. We use diet to focus on fuel, performance, emotion, social connection, and overall well being. They use diet for you to follow their rules. We use diet for you to create your own rules. They use diet to project their standards onto you. We use diet to achieve the standards you set for yourself. They use diet to make you feel like you're broken. We use diet to make you feel whole.

Let's reclaim that word and understand that when we look at the personality diet, it's a process for becoming the best version of you. It's breaking free of the current system that ignores individual differences. It's being able to achieve all of your goals and all of the results that you could ever want.

CHAPTER 3

PERSONALITY TYPES

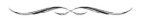

In this chapter, I'm going to go over the process for which we determine personality profiles, and how we use that information to build a protocol that allows for greater adherence and sustainability. This is a fluid process but we've been able to create something called the personality diet solution to go through a questionnaire, figure out what type of person you are, then dig a little bit deeper in understanding your experiences, your lifestyle, your current habits, your mindset, and what you're trying to accomplish to build a fully customizable plan that allows for success within your life and accounts for flexibility for all the things that are meaningful to you. This makes the process more enjoyable, more sustainable, and allows you to see the results you've been craving.

When we look at different personality types, we break this down into five profiles. Now, the important thing to understand before we get into each profile is that most people will have characteristics of many different profiles. This is not me saying that there are only five different people in the world. This is the way that we've found to be the most effective. You'll see that you have characteristics of multiple profiles, but you're always going to have one dominant personality type. You'll start to understand the connection between your dominant personality profile and why that matters from an adherence standpoint, from a lifestyle standpoint, and how it impacts your training and nutrition.

This has been studied by psychologists for a long time. There are many psychologists and neuroscientists who have connected personality traits with activity in different regions of the brain. For instance, if we look at something like fearfulness, that's typically linked to the amygdala and the pursuit of pleasure. So it's something that would be strongly connected with the neurotransmitter dopamine, which is basically our pleasure seeking neurotransmitter. Now, as a basic understanding of neurotransmitters, they're simply chemical messengers that deliver messages throughout our body and they control everything from our feelings and emotions to motor coordination and motor learning, to digestion, to feelings of pleasure, to fear and anxiety. There is not a single process that happens in the body without neurotransmitters. I like to think of them as little mailmen and mail women just delivering mail and messages all throughout the body. When we look at the connection between neurotransmitters and personalities, we can look at the pleasure system using dopamine. We also have a fearfulness system that's strongly connected to serotonin.

Serotonin activity is often associated with agreeableness and anxiety levels, it's kind of like that sense of well-being neurotransmitters. The higher levels of serotonin, the higher sense of well-being and contentment. Some people even refer to it as the happiness neurotransmitter. When we see an individual with low levels of serotonin, they're typically going to have higher levels of anxiety. We can actually look at your personality traits and gain insight into the neurotransmitter balance in your body. So we get to see and understand your brain chemistry, the way that you're wired. By looking at your personality traits, we know what neurotransmitter systems are dominant and what neurotransmitter systems are sensitive. Having that information allows us to apply certain practices that will align with your personality. Think of it like knowing your Love Language but in terms of fitness and nutrition. An example would be somebody who is dopamine dominant, which means that they are highly motivated by that pleasure-seeking neurotransmitter. That person would typically be more extroverted, they would be more of a risk taker. They would be the type of person who would want to drive a motorcycle 200 miles per hour or jump out of a plane because the dopamine response is so strong and their body is so sensitive to dopamine, they want to do that activity more and more. That's also why they're more prone to addiction and addictive-like behaviors. They're potentiated by any increase in dopamine so when they do an activity that stimulates a dopamine response, they can easily become addicted to that activity and want to do it more and more and at even greater levels of intensity over time. They're risk takers. They're very talkative. They're confrontational, more like a vocal leader. They take up a lot of space both physically and verbally. If we were to set up a protocol for that person, it wouldn't make sense to give them a boring, linear plan that's very cookie-cutter and methodical. We want to engage and appeal to their dopamine dominance. We want to cater to their competitive nature and their intense personality. It would look very different for the type of person who has low levels of serotonin. A person that is going to have higher anxiety. They require more structure. They require more organization, Somebody who has low levels of serotonin, they're going to be like your typical planners. They're going to be very practical and logical in the way that they think and in the way that they operate. It makes sense to give them as much information as we can and plan very strategically. We want to keep things very organized for that person. Anything new or anything that creates a novelty response is going to drive their anxiety up even higher, which is the last thing we want. That's why they crave organization, structure, and repetition. They need to feel safe and in total control due to their low levels of serotonin and higher levels of anxiety.

If we think about what people normally do, they look at all of these different protocols out there and try a lot of different things. If you're anything like me, your diet history has a laundry list of programs and meal plans like paleo, or keto or whole 30, or intermittent fasting or tracking macros. The number one question is, are those things right for you? That is what we have to understand. That's why we're using your personality to assess whether these different protocols are right for you and we can actually create something that is based on who you are as a person. When we look at all of the frustration that you've had in the past and feeling like you couldn't sustain what protocol you were doing, it wasn't your fault. You were just playing against a stacked deck.

When we understand the psychology of behavior change, and we understand how to make the process more sustainable based on your personality traits, all of a sudden things become much easier and more effective.

When we break down the personality profiles, we break it down into five descriptions. We have a confident vocal leader, who is someone with high self-esteem. They're going to be very talkative, very loud, very competitive. They don't do well with authority. They like to do things on their own terms. They love to argue. They're also going to be very charismatic, they're going to be more of a risk taker and have addictive personality traits. Those are the people who might be more prone to drug addiction or alcohol abuse because those things play on your dopamine receptors. They're not going to care what other people think of them. They are who they are and they don't care what you think. They're also going to be very impatient.

Now, when we look at the neurotransmitter balance in that person, they're going to typically have low levels of dopamine at rest, but they're going to be highly sensitive to dopamine. That means that any increase, anything that spikes dopamine, is going to cause a greater response and potentiation within that individual. Which means they're more likely to do that activity. In other words, taking a risk, getting into a fight, arguing, winning, competing, etc is because of their dopamine system. They are future-based thinkers. Motivated by the potential reward or pleasure response that they will get from an activity, even if it's a high-risk activity. Keeping adequate dopamine levels and maintaining dopamine sensitivity is extremely important. That can be accomplished through a nutritious diet, regular exercise, quality sleep, stress management, and avoiding high dopamine spikes from things like drugs, alcohol, high sugar meals, highly processed foods, blue lights, excess video games, social media, or TV. These individuals are also going to be better at handling stress because of their high levels of inhibitory neurotransmitters. We have neurotransmitters that are responsible for calming us down and slowing brain activity. When we look at anxiety, it's nothing more than an increase in neuronal activity. Meaning your neurons are firing so fast that it is creating very real scenarios in your head that's making you anxious. The neurotransmitters that are responsible for slowing down that brain activity are serotonin and GABA. Our confident vocal leader, they typically have very high levels of both serotonin and GABA, which allows them to recover better from any sort of stress. They're the person that likes to burn the candle at both ends because they can handle more stress and have intense personalities. These are the factors that we need to consider when we're talking about a diet plan or training approach for that individual. Their training needs to be structured in a way for them to "win" each workout. We want to engage that intense personality. They do well by lifting heavier, adding more weight to the bar, and getting stronger in the gym. Within their nutrition, we want them to see early results. Because they're so competitive, a long and methodical plan will disengage them.

They'll think they can do it better on their own. We want to get quick results on the front end to cater to their personality type and get them to buy in to the process. Since we know they can handle more stress, we typically can get a little more aggressive with our approach for this individual. They already have higher levels of inhibitory neurotransmitters that calm the brain down. And carbs are a great way to increase inhibitory neurotransmitters, particularly serotonin, to help lower stress. However, since they already have higher levels of serotonin and GABA, a lower carb plan can work well for this particular personality type.

Do you have a friend that always needs to be right? Or maybe it's you. You know that person who will argue anything and everything just to prove they're right? They even have the amazing ability to argue and convince you that they're right, even if you're agreeing with them! They're the type of person who walks into a room and takes control and command right away. They have the ability to just be who they are and say what's on their mind and they don't care if you like it or not. Do you know that person? That's the personality type we're talking about when we're discussing the confident, vocal leader.

Then we have the imaginative leader by example, and they're going to have very similar traits to the confident vocal leader. However, the biggest difference is that they're not going to be as competitive or as intense. They also are dopamine dominant. They're also motivated by that reward response in the brain. So it's also important for this individual that we take the same precautions in keeping dopamine levels adequate and maintaining dopamine sensitivity. However, they have more of an explosive personality. They're more creative and imaginative and the reason is that they have higher levels of acetylcholine, which is the neurotransmitter that's responsible for motor learning and brain communication. If you're trying to learn a new skill, having high levels of acetylcholine is incredibly important so they're naturally athletic and fast learners. They're going to be typical multi-taskers. They like to try new things. They pick up things very quickly. They're more goal-oriented. They're more like your dreamers. They perform very well under pressure. They're very impatient. They need that mental stimulation because high levels of acetylcholine mean that you like to do a lot of things at once. They're the people that seemingly can multitask very well and don't seem distracted by doing a bunch of things at once. Multitasking is actually not something that we can do. The appearance of multitasking is having the ability to switch attention from one task to the next so fast that it gives off the impression of multitasking. Acetylcholine speeds up the brain communication process which is why these individuals appear so good at multitasking. So they need that mental stimulation, otherwise, they'll get very bored. As you can imagine, if we set that person up on a nutrition plan that doesn't require much thinking, that doesn't challenge them, that just kind of goes through the motions, they're going to lose motivation very quickly. We want to cater to who they are as a person to allow for greater adherence and more enjoyment. Knowing the personality traits is such a huge advantage in this process. This personality type also has high levels of the inhibitory neurotransmitters, serotonin, and GABA. To understand the difference, GABA calms and relaxes the brain, whereas serotonin helps with impulse control, pain relief, and influences a positive mood. These individuals can also handle a higher amount of stress so they also do well with more of an aggressive approach to nutrition and can also do well with a lower carb plan. When it comes to training, they enjoy training in line with their personality, which is more explosive by nature. They like fast movements that require more brain activation. Do you have that friend that always seems to pick things up quickly? They're naturally athletic and it just seems like they learn new skills almost effortlessly. The person that leads by example, is usually the star athlete for their team, and can explode from 0 to 100 and back to 0 in almost an instant. That's who we're talking about when we discuss the imaginative leader by example.

Then as we move along, we have the social chameleon, who is a typical people pleaser. They can adapt to any situation and can change their personality based on the environment that they're in. They're great at reading people as a way of being adaptive and fitting into almost any situation. They know what to do to get the reciprocity that they crave. They're indecisive and they're procrastinators. That's because they want to be liked by everyone. So, if this person wants to choose a restaurant and they're going out with a group of people, they're going to be afraid that they're decision will not be liked by everyone. So it makes them indecisive. They hate to feel left out. They need constant change and variation. They get bored very quickly. They want to keep things fresh and will often leave tasks undone just to move on to something new. They typically go all-in on a new task that they love, but they often lose interest very quickly and move to the next thing. They perform better when they're up against a deadline. The opinion of others is very important to them. The reason for all of this is that they are adrenaline dominant. Now, many people know of adrenaline as the neurotransmitter that's responsible for the stress response in the body. These individuals are very sensitive to adrenaline. So oftentimes they can seem like two totally different people were at rest, they can be more introverted, calmer, more relaxed, but the minute that adrenaline increases, the minute they're in a stressful situation, it's like they become this alpha version of themselves. It's like the adrenaline takes over. That could be anything from being out at a bar or listening to music and dancing or going out to a party or even working out. Training and exercise increase adrenaline so that person might be way more confident in the gym than they are just lounging at home. With understanding this need for variation, understanding the adrenaline sensitivity of this individual, we can then begin to incorporate different strategies within their nutrition and training to allow for greater adherence and enjoyment. Their neurological makeup is such that they have low levels of adrenaline at rest, high sensitivity to any increase in adrenaline, and a well-balanced profile of all the other neurotransmitters. Which is why their behavior is very adaptive. The low levels of adrenaline typically mean they're more insecure when they're not in a stressful situation. The elevation in adrenaline will give them more confidence which is why they perform better when they're up against a deadline and that makes them procrastinators. Their ability to read people really well is also a survival mechanism based on their neurotransmitter balance. When an individual is insecure, they want to get assurance that other people like them. However, it's not good enough to

31

just hear it, they need to see it and believe it. So they develop a sense for reading people to know if other people like them and they crave that reciprocity. These individuals will do anything for the respect, admiration, and approval of others. Even developing different personas to fit in with specific groups of people or social circles. It can even come across as fake but it's just part of their nature. Often times these individuals make great actors. When it comes to training and nutrition, we want to cater to their need for variation. The reason they love novelty so much is that it stimulates an adrenaline response. Once a task becomes routine or repetitive, they no longer get the adrenaline they crave and they lose interest very quickly. That's why these individuals are classic program hoppers. So there's a balancing act that needs to happen. We want to keep variation in the mix but we also want them to make progress. We know that jumping from program to program makes it challenging to see progress in the long term. Therefore, we want to give them new things to try while intelligently progressing them through the process. An example might be, having them progress through a training program but using different metabolic finishers to keep things fresh. Or having them progress through their nutrition but using calorie cycling or carb cycling for 3-4 week blocks, then switching the method for another 3-4 week block to keep that variety in the mix, while also progressing them in an intelligent manner. From a neurological standpoint, we want to maintain adequate levels of dopamine because adrenaline is fabricated downstream from dopamine. Therefore, to have enough resources to produce adrenaline, we want to make sure that dopamine levels do not get too low. We also want to maintain adrenaline sensitivity, which is extremely important for this individual. The adrenergic receptors can actually desensitize very quickly so this is something to be aware of. This is a simple survival mechanism that makes sense from an evolutionary standpoint. Adrenaline is kind of like the NOS in your car. It's produced to handle a stressful situation that may be life or death. We evolved to handle acute stress due to being faced with predators and a constant battle for survival. There were not many chronic stressors thousands of years ago. Therefore, adrenaline is part of our sympathetic nervous system response, which is our fight or flight mode. All things normal, it should elevate for a short period of time while we fight or flee from the stress, and then return to baseline. As such, the adrenergic receptors can desensitize if adrenaline stays attached to the receptors for a long period of time or if adrenaline is overproduced due to chronic stress. Proper stress management, nutrition, training, sleep, and lifestyle factors are important for this individual.

Do you know that person who can adjust their behavior and personality in any situation? They have a hard time making decisions because they don't want to let anyone down. They are classic people pleasers and would do anything for the approval of others. That's the type of person we're referring to when we talk about social chameleons.

Next, we have the profile that I call the emotional supporter. This is somebody who is like your best friend in a one on one situation. Everything that they do is driven by emotion and driven by feel. That is because their dominant neurotransmitter is glutamate. And glutamate is responsible for some of our memory, but it is also our emotional amplifier. So if you have a feeling and emotion plus high levels of glutamate, that emotional response is going to be amplified. Instead of just feeling happy, you feel euphoric. Instead of feeling sad, you feel depressed. These are the people that are glutamate dominant. They need to feel important. They're great listeners. They fall in love very easily. They give all of themselves to others. They're very empathetic but they also have higher anxiety and have a more difficult time saying no because they hate to disappoint people. They make their decisions based off of emotion, feeling, and instinct. They are the most likely of the profiles to emotionally eat or binge eat. The interesting thing about glutamate when we look at how it's connected to emotional eating and a strong neurological response to food, and we'll go over this more in-depth in a future chapter, but glutamate has been added to foods by engineers to increase your emotional response to that food. It's mostly been added to fast food, frozen meals, commercial coffee in the form of MSG or l-glutamic acid.

Imagine you just ate a fast-food burger. You'll get a dopamine spike from that burger, so there's a pleasure response that happens, but there's also glutamate added to that food. The internal drive that you will feel to want to eat that again is going to be much higher. You have this strong pleasure response along with a strong emotional response of euphoria from that food. It's playing on your brain chemistry, and remember that food engineers are brilliant at what they do. They get paid a lot of money to make foods hyper-palatable and easy to overeat. So they're playing on your neurological systems in order to get you to over-consume and want to eat that food again and again. You end up having a strong connection to that burger and you'll want to try that burger again. Recently, studies have come out showing that excess levels of glutamate can be neurotoxic and can have some neurodegenerative effects. It can be toxic to the brain, which has forced more strict regulations on managing glutamate added to foods, which is a good thing. But it's something to be aware of when you find yourself having addictive-like behaviors towards specific foods. Oftentimes, the reason is that it's playing on your brain chemistry. It's playing on your dopaminergic system and circulating glutamate levels. It's especially something to be aware of with this particular personality type. The emotional supporter also has low levels of GABA, which as we know, is the neurotransmitter that calms down the brain. This is the reason for their higher levels of anxiety. Being more emotionally driven, and having higher anxiety, leads to these individuals being very hard on themselves. They have the tendency to beat themselves up and will often shut down if they feel they've let someone down, especially a loved one or mentor. These individuals crave positive reinforcement and want to know that they've done a good job. That's why they like to train in a way that provides that positive reinforcement. Feeling that muscle soreness or having a pool of sweat on the floor for this personality type can be very motivating. It's that direct feedback to them that they've done a good job and accomplished something. This is why they gravitate towards training that emphasizes feel, mind-muscle connection, a great muscle pump, but also training that makes them sweat and feel accomplished like a spin class or orange theory class. When it comes to their nutrition, moderation is typically the best approach. The reason is that glutamate can be increased when carb consumption is high. Having a high carb plan will increase their levels of glutamate even further which can cause some issues for this personality type. However, we also know that carbs can help increase inhibitory neurotransmitters, particularly serotonin, so a low carb plan can increase their anxiety even further. Interestingly enough, a keto diet can actually increase GABA but decrease serotonin so it may be helpful as a temporary solution but the long term can be harmful for this individual. Ultimately, a moderate carb approach and balanced nutrition, with an emphasis on food quality is the best way to go for this person. Too much processed food and their glutamate levels will increase even more. It's important for this individual to incorporate lifestyle practices and habits to increase GABA. For example, having a sound sleep routine, eating quality foods, incorporating mindfulness practices, stress management, and keeping their circadian rhythm uninterrupted.

You know that person who is so easy to talk to because they're such a great listener? The individual who would give you the shirt off their back. They seem to fall in love easily and really appreciate grand gestures, dressing up nicely, and pour all of themselves into their romantic relationships. The person that is really hard on themselves and when things aren't going well, you know it because you don't hear from them. That's who we're talking about when we discuss the emotional supporter.

Lastly, we have an organized planner. This is somebody like the example I gave earlier, who has low levels of serotonin. They're naturally more anxious. They're more of a perfectionist. A planner. They're very practical, analytical, and they prefer repetition over novelty. Because if you

36

have a low sense of well-being with higher anxiety, then something new is going to cause tension and uncertainty. This person wants to follow a plan. They're very patient. They don't like to take risks. They want structure and rules. They don't like to talk about themselves very much. They're more introverted. They're very focused and detail oriented.

Now, when they master a skill, which is something that they love to do, they're technical masters, then they can become very confident in what they're doing. So they can accomplish anything but want to feel in total control first. Throwing them into a new situation will just drive their anxiety up even more. Once they get to a point where they've mastered something, which could be in their work life or fitness, they become more confident and proficient. But before that, they're going to be somebody who operates with a little bit more anxiety and reservedness. This individual also doesn't feel the need to change or modify their behavior to fit in. They are who they are and typically don't care what others think. There's a lot we can do from a lifestyle, training, and nutrition perspective to help them get the results they want. We can get them to a place of feeling in total control and increased confidence. From a training standpoint, we want to give them a chance to master and feel in control of every movement. They don't need variation and actually do better with more repetition and practice. These individuals gravitate towards more endurance activities like running or cycling. When it comes to nutrition, we also want to give them a very organized, detailed, and structured plan. Due to their low levels of serotonin, this personality type does very well on a higher carb plan because carbs will increase serotonin. A helpful process for this individual is to establish as much of a routine in their day to day life as possible. We also know that these individuals are prone to having higher levels of cortisol, which is our stress hormone. Cortisol often gets a bad rap, but it's often misguided. It's a necessary hormone and does a lot of good things in the body like mobilizing stored energy to prepare us for stressful events. However, issues arise when cortisol is chronically elevated. This can cause a lower metabolic rate, more prone to sickness, chronic fatigue, and a number of other issues. That's why we want to have plenty of stress management practices in place for this personality type. Getting outside in natural light in the morning, going for walks, meditating, journaling, avoiding blue lights close to bedtime, doing hobbies you enjoy, prioritizing sleep, and having a proper training and nutrition protocol in place will be extremely important for this individual. You know that person who never really likes to talk about themselves? The person who is naturally more anxious. They are not swayed by emotions and make decisions based on logic and information. This individual is incredibly organized and loves to follow a plan. That's who we're talking about when we talk about the organized planner.

When we look at the five personality profiles, those are the descriptions and the characteristics and why it's so important. Knowing your personality type gives us insight into your neurotransmitter balance which is basically a way of saying, how your brain is wired. That provides us a lot of information on how we should establish a protocol for better adherence and sustainability. That is the exact process that we take everyone through which we call the personality diet solution. We start with a neurological optimization phase, which will improve your mood stability, sense of well being, and motivation. Then we set the framework for the individual variables in your life. Again, we have to dig into your lifestyle, the way your schedule is set up, your personal preferences, your history, your goals, your mindset, etc. That allows us to create a protocol that you will enjoy and that will produce the results that you want.

CHAPTER 4

THE ULTIMATE KEYS TO SUCCESS

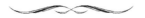

I'm probably going to sound like a broken record here, but the ultimate keys to long term success are adherence and sustainability. Now, when we look at adherence and sustainability at the root of all dieting, this is why most people fail. It's because they can't adhere to or sustain what they're doing. We talked about this earlier but remember that the way most diets are set up, is to have you follow a certain set of rules without factoring in who you are as an individual. What happens is that maybe you follow along for a short period of time, and maybe see some short term success, but we know that true change takes time. Therefore, if you can't adhere to and sustain what you're doing, those results are going to be short-lived. I want to use a practical example because keto is very popular right now, so I'm going to use that as an example but this is not me picking on keto. There is nothing inherently wrong with a ketogenic diet. When I say keto, I'm not talking about a medical application of keto, I'm talking about a very low-carb to no-carb plan.

A lot of people use this as a way to quickly achieve some form of weight loss. There are people who are successful with it because they don't actually enjoy eating carbs and it becomes a lifestyle. However, studies show that the long term compliance for a ketogenic diet is extremely low. Most people fail at the ketogenic diet long term because it is unrealistic to eliminate carbs from their life. What happens is they do it for a short period of time, but then life gets in the way. Maybe they want to go out to eat with their family. And of course, when you go out there's going to be bread served at the table, there's going to be carbs with every meal, and all of a sudden it becomes really challenging to navigate life without eating carbohydrates. This is where one slip up can lead to that dangerous slope of all or nothing dieting. The type of mindset where you feel like, well, I messed up my diet, so now I'm going to eat all the carbs I possibly can because they're going to be taken away from me very soon. This comes back to that last chance syndrome where you want to eat as much as you can of the food that is "off-limits." Then what happens is they'll start back at square one. They'll eliminate carbs again and go through this process over and over. Oftentimes, they'll end up worse than when they started.

This concept is not unique to just keto or low carb dieting. There was a 2005 study that looked at 4 popular dietary protocols to determine which diet, if any, was best. The study looked at low carb, zone, weight watchers, and the Ornish diet. What the researchers found was that all diets produced the same or similar results when properly adhered to. Therefore, there was no one diet that was better than the others. The determining factor was simply - adherence.

41

So when we look at the ultimate keys to success, we have to start with adherence and sustainability. Can you do what you're doing for the rest of your life? This helps explain why some methods work for some people but fail miserably for others. Maybe you've been a part of a fitness community or you've paid attention to what your co-workers are doing or a family member, and you want to try what they're doing because they've seen great success with a certain diet. There's nothing inherently wrong with that. However, you have to understand that what works for them is not necessarily going to work for you because they are individuals and have their own unique needs. Their metabolism is different, their lifestyle is different, their personal preferences are different, their personality traits are different. So to look at what they're doing, and try to apply it to yourself, typically doesn't end well. Again, it just comes back to understanding your individual goals, what is sustainable for your lifestyle, and what you can adhere to the most effectively and effortlessly.

When we look at the goal of a successful diet, in reality, it's to not feel like you're dieting. It's to actually enjoy the process and feel like you can do exactly what you're doing for the rest of your life. That doesn't mean there won't be any sort of challenge or discipline involved. Because there will be. Anything worth changing is going to require some form of effort and hardship. If it wasn't challenging, it wouldn't be worth it. I don't want to make it seem like it's all smooth sailing but the point is that when we look at the big picture, you shouldn't feel like you have to overhaul everything in your life just to fit within your dietary protocol. I remember something from my personal journey when I was doing a meal plan that had a food list that I was allowed to eat and a food list that I wasn't allowed to eat. During that time of my life, I would avoid going out with my friends and I would avoid seeing my family. I knew I was going to be put in positions where I'd be surrounded by those foods that were off-limits. My solution was to just stay home by myself. Literally eating chicken and broccoli, thinking that I was doing it in the name of health. I would have friends who would go out and when they would invite me, I would have to make an excuse. I would say that I was sick and that I couldn't make it. I would lie to my friends and family, all for the sake of staying on my diet.

Now, that doesn't seem like the healthiest relationship with food. But at the time, I didn't realize it. I just thought that I was making these choices because it was better for my health and that's a very narrow, very short-sighted focus because when we look at health, it's an all encompassing sphere. We can't just segment different parts of our health. Our physical health is only one singular component. We have to look at our connections with people, our relationships, life experiences, emotional health, mental health, spiritual health. It is truly all encompassing. There are certain times where the best thing you can do for your health is to connect with somebody that you love. Maybe that means sharing a slice of pizza and a glass of wine, even though it's not serving your physical health at that exact moment. It is serving another part of your health that is equally as important. So when we look at our dietary protocols, we shouldn't have to overhaul everything in our life just to fit within these rules that have been placed upon us. I lost out on some meaningful connections because of the choices that I made to adhere to my diet at the time. Experiences that I'll

43

never get back. There is a lot of research on what helps people live longer. Research on areas of the world called Blue Zones, which are where some of the longest living people reside. The interesting thing is when we look at Blue Zones, which have the largest population of people who live beyond 100, is that their nutrition is all over the place. There are not many consistencies amongst the different nutrition protocols from different Blue Zone regions. Some of them have diets that are higher in carbs. Some of them have diets that are higher in fats. One thing is that most of the groups eat a lot of vegetables, which makes sense. However, everything else is kind of unique to that area. But what we do see is that they have a strong sense of community. They are more active, they walk more, they have better relationships, stronger one on one relationships, and stronger connections to each other. They're naturally more active with things like walking and lower intensity activities. When we talk about health, we really have to factor in some of those other variables like your life experiences, how you're able to connect with people, the relationships in your life. And if your diet is removing you from those situations where you can't foster that area of your health, it is doing more harm than good. I don't care what the nutrient value of your diet is at that point. If it is requiring you to avoid your friends and to avoid your family, then it is doing more harm than good. Something that I take a lot of pride in when we look at the personality diet, is the lifestyle component. It's the impact that it's had on our clients, beyond just fitness and nutrition. I thought it would be a powerful thing to show you some of the success stories we've had from clients who chimed in with one or two sentences about what the personality diet has meant for them.

-*Season* commented "the personality diet has meant empowerment. Trust in myself and the confident knowledge that I can achieve my goals."

-*Danny* said that "the personality diet has meant actually teaching me to enjoy the journey while living my best life."

-*Gina* said that "it means accepting my choices and the flexibility that I have in my life."

-*Jan* says "it has empowered me to learn to listen to and love the body I have been gifted and to maximize my choices for healthy aging."

-*Kate* says that "the personality diet is teaching me that I can enjoy life and still crush my goals."

-*Nicole* said that "it means freedom from perfection."

-*Danielle* says that "it has taught me that being consistent is not synonymous with being perfect and that I can achieve my goals without being someone else's textbook definition of perfect. It has also taught me that all the knowledge of nutrition and fitness in the world is nothing without the mindset."

-*Sherry* says "it has taught me that I am not broken. We all have our own path to our own goals. And it is not a straight line to get there. mindset, patience and consistency win."

-*Becky* says that "it's more than nutrition, it's a life-transforming experience."

-*Jennifer* says that "the personality diet has had a tremendous impact on my physical and mental health. I've gotten more progress in three months than I've had in approximately two years with another company."

-*Erin* says that "it has taught me to trust myself to listen when I feel like something is off and when I'm feeling good. It has also taught me the freedom to make my own choices and priorities."

-*Ronnie* says that "the personality diet allows for the power to make the choices best for forward movement at your own pace."

-*Erica* says that "it taught me that my journey is so much more than just physical change and that being successful doesn't mean being perfect."

-*Hope* says that "it's realistic and positive support of a healthy mind and body."

-*Melissa* says that "it has meant body composition improvements, even through vacation enjoying awesome foods through multiple holiday gatherings, work travel, date nights, coffee creamer, dinner with friends, ice cream, and even vodka."

-*KeithAnn* said that "it has meant freedom and understanding. I feel more like myself than I have for a long time and I have the freedom and support to embrace that I have the freedom to live life and know that I have control over my body, to overcome whatever weight/nutrition challenges that come up, which stems from understanding. The change in anxiety surrounding my body and food is life changing."

-*Jessica* says that "it has meant to me that there's nothing wrong with me. It taught me self-love."

-*Lori* says that "it has given me the flexibility to still be me while learning how to push the limits of what I thought was possible."

-*Theresa* says that "it's a way of life to live happy and healthy and has led me to exceed any and all of my goals and it isn't over yet."

-*Sherry* says that "it has taught me to be inflexible about the goals I choose, but flexible about the method to get there."

-*Erica* said, "I don't need to be perfect for things to be effective. The plan just needs to be right for me." Billi says that "it has meant simply freedom."

-*Rachel* said that it's given her self-esteem, self-worth, and self-love.

-*Colleen* says "the personality diet to me has given me the knowledge to figure out who I am and how to get to where I want to be physically and mentally."

-*Wanda* says that "it has helped make an ally of myself. I know what I need, what I enjoy and what is sustainable."

-*Sarah* says that "it has helped me realize that I'm able to find balance and that I'm able and I'm capable of reaching my goals."

-Kristen says "it has given me a chance to feel like myself again. I've developed a healthier mindset, a chance to figure out what my path is and why I want this path, feeling less guilt about my choices and learning that consistency will guide me to my success and it takes time and patience."

-And *AZ* says that "it is a change in mindset. So you can keep training, eating and living life the way that you want consistently, to achieve all of your goals and those three assets of your life."

As you can see, the impact of focusing on who you are as a person and finding a way that is sustainable for you truly has a profound impact. The cool thing about all of those testimonials is that each and every one of those protocols looks completely different. They are unique to the individual. They factor in who they are as a person, their personality traits, their individual variables that allow for that feeling of freedom. It has provided a lifelong solution for each of those individuals. More importantly, that is just a small percentage and a small insight into the change that we are creating and the movement that we are leading. The personality diet solution is changing the standard in the industry as a whole.

CHAPTER 5

GROWTH VERSUS FIXED MINDSET

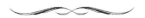

The word mindset is a bit of a buzzword right now that gets thrown around in fitness circles and there's actually a lot of validity to it, although I'm not sure a lot of the people who talk about mindset actually know what they're talking about. When we talk about mindset, we're simply discussing our perceptions and perspectives in how we view and interpret situations. Your mindset is your own personal lens that allows you to form thoughts, decisions, beliefs, and values. The idea of growth versus fixed mindset is a concept that was made popular by Carol Dweck, in which she stated that mindset exists on a continuum from fixed to growth with regards to how we view our own abilities, skills, and attributes. It's important to understand that mindset is a fluid and dynamic spectrum. Therefore, it's possible (and likely) that you will have a growth mindset in certain areas of your life and a fixed mindset in others. The cool thing about having a growth mindset is that it's actually a strong predictor for your ability to change. Countless studies have shown that a growth mindset is predictive of success in many areas, including weight loss. We also know that having a growth mindset about health and fitness is strongly correlated with actively practicing more health-promoting behaviors. Therefore, anytime we're trying to make a change in our lifestyle, our behavior, or our habits, we can look directly at our mindset and the belief that we have in ourselves. This will be a strong predictor for our ability to make that change. This applies directly to health and fitness, but it also applies to your career path, your relationships, and many other areas of your life.

One of the best ways to elicit a growth mindset in an area of your life that you're trying to improve upon is to draw on current examples where you already have a growth mindset. For example, if you've been able to exhibit a growth mindset with your ability to learn a new language or play an instrument, we can draw from that experience and help apply that to your fitness and nutrition. The first step in this process is to create awareness around your fixed mindset and then we can seek to actively change it. Some signs of having a fixed mindset are avoiding challenging or difficult things, giving up easily, viewing failure as proof that you're not good enough, being threatened by others who succeed, believing your abilities are innate, and frequently thinking "why bother." The good news is that there are practices we can implement to move from a fixed mindset to more of a growth mindset. Before we get deeper into growth versus fixed mindset, we have to look at just what is a mindset as a whole.

As I mentioned, it's most easily classified as the belief about ourselves or about the world around us. Therefore, if you interpret your ability to make a change as something you have little control over like you were just dealt this hand, that's going to be a very fixed mindset. The feeling and belief that you can't change certain characteristics or attributes about yourself. For example, maybe you believe that your genetics are the determining factor for your ability to lose weight so you don't even bother trying because you feel like it's out of your control. Those with more of a growth mindset believe that they can improve, that they can get better with the right practice and the right effort so that nothing is set in stone, even though they may understand that they're just not good at something yet. They believe that eventually, they can get there.

For example, somebody who wants to write a book might be very well aware that they're not a good writer yet but they know that through practice, repetition, and learning, they can get better and get to the point where they write a book successfully. Having a growth mindset will greatly improve your ability to create a successful transformation when it comes to your health and fitness. If someone has a fixed mindset, they'll use their preexisting beliefs about themselves as reasons to prevent them from making sustainable change. When somebody has a growth mindset about their fitness, they will view their ability to learn and create change as something that is well within their control. Therefore, they will view any setbacks that they have as learning opportunities. They don't view it as proof that they're a failure, they view it as an opportunity to learn and get better. It's the difference between viewing the hand that you're dealt with and using it to play the victim, versus looking at the situation as a puzzle that needs to be figured out. Each setback simply means that we have to rearrange the puzzle, then figure out the best path forward. A real-life example would be in the form of self-restraint. If an individual has more of a growth mindset, they're going to be better equipped to handle situations where their willpower or discipline is tested. Let's use the example that many people experience in the workplace where there are always treats and candy available in the break room. The growth-minded individual believes in their ability to make a change. So they're more likely to realize that the choice to pass on treats or candy is within their control. A fixed mindset individual is more likely to grab the candy from the bowl, and even though they have a goal to achieve better health, they may say something like, I just can't resist the candy bowl. Almost like it wasn't their decision. That's a very fixed mindset. That individual is less likely to achieve the results that they want over time because they don't believe in their ability to change their behaviors or actions. This is why it's so critical to be aware of your fixed mindset tendencies and then actively working to move to a growth mindset over time. We can look at this in terms of what the research says and show examples of how improving your mindset from fixed to growth will have a profound impact on your ability to see success within every area of your life.

I want to talk about research that was conducted at Columbia University. They found that the people who believed that they could increase their intelligence got better grades and test scores in school. It was a simple study that illustrated one's belief in becoming more intelligent, allowing them to score better on tests and get better grades. We can apply that information to the fitness world. There was a study done by scientists at North Carolina State University who wanted to see that exact process unfold. They wanted to test how the belief in your ability to get healthier and change your exercise behavior would impact your results.

117 people answered a bunch of questions about their mindset regarding exercise and their ability to become a more fit individual. They also asked them questions about their exercise habits. The research found that those who had more of a growth mindset in regards to fitness reported exercising more frequently in the past compared to those with a more fixed mindset. This study was based on analyzing the naturally occurring mindset in those individuals, which confirms what we already know. Some people are just naturally wired more than others to engage in health promoting behaviors. However, the interesting question is, what if we could change that perception? What if we could take those who had a naturally more fixed mindset and transition them into more of a growth mindset?

Let's look at another study where they randomly assigned 156 women and 158 men and had them either read an article about the changeable nature of fitness or an article that was focused on how your genetics impair your ability to become more fit. So one of the articles was more of a growth mindset article that talked about the changeable nature of your fitness. The other article was more of a fixed mindset article that talked about how your genetics pre-determine your ability to become more fit. The researchers had everyone answer a bunch of questions in the beginning of the study and at the end of the study about their mindset and their exercise habits. In order to prevent the subjects from realizing what the study was intended to do, they deceived them about the purpose of the articles. They asked them to provide feedback about the comprehensibility before it was used in another study. That way, the subjects believed they were simply providing feedback regarding the articles and wouldn't be aware of the intended purpose. What the researchers found was that the simple task of reading an article dramatically influenced the individual's mindset. The people that read the article about the possibility of improving their health and fitness were reported as having much stronger growth mindsets on the questionnaire. And those who read the article that the nature of their fitness was all tied to their genetics scored much lower on the mindset questionnaire, so their mindset was more fixed. The interesting part was that the effect was observed despite their initial mindset. In other words, somebody who came in with more of a fixed mindset was able to develop more of a growth mindset after reading one single article about the ability to improve their fitness. On the other side, the people who naturally had a growth mindset ended up with more of a fixed mindset after reading this one single article about the inability to improve their fitness. The question then, is that even though their mindset's changed, can this be something to establish a long term mindset difference? Or is it just an acute effect?

There's a lot of research that still needs to be done. However, we have these simple interventions that we know will improve mindset. We know that those with a stronger growth mindset are more likely to engage in health promoting behaviors. We also know that if we can take someone from a fixed to growth mindset that the likelihood of them engaging in more health promoting behaviors is greater. Therefore, we can apply these

54

short term interventions and use them to create more self-belief which is going to be paramount in creating change.

There's another study that was done at Washington State University, where the researchers sent 34 women and 39 men through a questionnaire about their mindset regarding body weight and then gave them a fake test with M&Ms and raisins. They were trying to use M&Ms as the "unhealthy" snack and the raisins as the "healthy" snack. The subjects were led to believe that the study was intended to get their feedback on the snacks themselves. Like a taste test that was being disguised as the true purpose of the study. In reality, they wanted to evaluate the mindsets about body weight and how that relates to the snacks that were consumed. What they found was that the people with a growth mindset ate fewer calories from M&Ms. The people that had a fixed mindset ate more.

They expected that mindset would play no role in the number of raisins consumed because less self-regulation is required to resist overeating raisins compared to M&Ms, and that was exactly what they found from the study. In other words, the subject's mindset didn't affect how many calories they ate of the "healthy" snack. However, those with a growth mindset were able to resist eating significantly more M&Ms than those with the fixed mindset. This makes sense if we break it down logically. If you believe that your dietary choices have little to no impact on your body weight because you have no control over creating change, then why would you regulate how much you eat of something like M&Ms. Your genetics are going to determine your fate anyway. On the flip side, if you believe in your ability to create change through your nutritional choices, then it makes sense that you just naturally resist over consuming something like M&Ms.

Your mindset plays an important role in your eating and your exercise behaviors without you even realizing it. Everything that we do with the personality diet first begins by creating awareness around some of these mindset hurdles. It's to bring to light some of the preconceived notions that you may have about yourself. Oftentimes we must unpack past experiences that are impacting your current behaviors. If you look at some of the neuroscience literature, you'll find that there's a strong connection between your mindset and the way that your brain operates. There was a study that was done at Michigan State University, where the researchers had participants wear an electrode cap to measure the electrical patterns in their brains while working through a complex task. Specifically, they were looking for areas of the brain related to attention to light up. Participants answered a question related to the task they were asked to complete. They were told if they answered correctly and then they were later told what the correct answer was. The researchers found that the attention part of the brain lit up differently depending on the mindset of the participant. People with a fixed mindset about intelligence only paid attention to whether their answer was right or wrong with little to no interest in the correct answer. Subjects with a growth mindset about intelligence wanted all of the information. They wanted to know whether their answer was right and if it was wrong, they wanted to know what the correct answer was. Again, just further reiterating the importance of mindset on your ability to make a change and seek out information to help you. Education is an important part of the process. The more that you can learn about healthy habits and nutrition, the more that you can create self-awareness, the more long term change you're going to be able to create. This is a huge asset in the sustainability factor that we talked about.

There are some practical takeaways from this understanding of the importance of our mindset as it relates to our likelihood of creating change. There are some things that we can do to cultivate a growth mindset. The first thing is being grateful for what you've accomplished so far, being okay with not being where you want to be quite yet. It's possible to love yourself exactly where you are right now and also actively seek improvement. Those two things aren't mutually exclusive. I talked about the example of somebody wanting to write a book and feeling like they're just not a good writer. With a growth mindset, you'll feel like I'm not where I need to be yet, but you'll believe you can get there. One of the things that we can do is just simply get started. As basic as it sounds, putting in the reps and seeing improvements happen over time is a huge asset. We can use past experiences to assist in our belief to get better in other areas. Think about something that you weren't good at in the past, and now quite proficient. Through practice and repetition, you achieved a better result and got better over time. We can use that experience to say, I'm not there yet, but I know I can get there. Putting in consistent reps is an important part of the process for fostering a growth mindset.

Another thing that can really help is finding someone who has accomplished what you want to accomplish and talk to them. Listening to somebody who has made a change, and listening to somebody who has a growth mindset can impact your mindset. This is why I'm a big believer in the power of community. Our Personality Diet community is one where we help each other in cultivating a growth mindset. We have people who have gone through a lot of different struggles, hardships, challenges, and setbacks. We use those as opportunities to learn and grow. When you have successful people around you, combined with social support, it's going to help you enforce more of a growth mindset.

Another tool we can utilize is journaling. Writing down why you want to be healthy and fit. Writing down the habits that you want to accomplish. Journal about the behavior change that you want to accomplish, your goals, your accomplishments, some of the obstacles you've overcome. Some strategies when journaling is to look at what you're trying to accomplish. Also, look at what you have already accomplished and practice gratitude for that. One thing that helps to put things in perspective is to write like you're giving advice to your best friend who's in your exact situation. What would you tell them? Then, apply that information to yourself. The bottom line is that we understand the importance of habits and behavior change in creating success within our health and fitness. We also know that our mindset is a great indicator of whether we will continue with that change or if we will give up on ourselves because of our internal beliefs. We can't separate the thoughts that we're having from our physical health or our emotional health. It's all connected. If we understand that, we can start to elicit more of a growth mindset, which will allow us to create habits and practices in our life to enhance our ability to create change. We can increase our likelihood of having a growth mindset and taking control of our own situation. Just remember that regardless of where you are in the process, you can continue to get better and you can increase that belief in yourself that you can create positive change.

CHAPTER 6

BEHAVIOR CHANGE

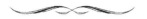

Before we get started on the specifics of how to change your behavior, I want to first mention that this is like everything else, a very individual process. There are many tactics and strategies you can use but everyone is different. Finding what works best for you is going to be key. What that means is that it might take some time and some trial and error, but truly, you need to be like a detective in finding the solution that works for you. It's important not to get frustrated. If one tactic doesn't work, it just means it's not the right fit for you. Similarly, like when we try a specific diet protocol and it doesn't work, that doesn't mean there's anything wrong with you, it just means it wasn't the right fit. There are still things that we can take away from that experience that we can then apply to future attempts. When you go through a diet program that doesn't work, learn about why that didn't work for you. What specifically did you not like about that process? What did you like? Maybe there were some positives that you can take away and apply to the next thing as you seek to create that lifelong solution.

It's the same thing with behavior change and creating healthy habits. We have to find what works for us as individuals. Now understanding the process for which behavior change takes place is an important way to get started. Understanding that when you have goals to accomplish, whether it's getting healthier, breaking a bad habit, whatever goals you want to achieve, we can help ourselves through this process by understanding the way that behavior change takes place. The first thing to assess is your readiness to make a change. Do you know why this is meaningful for you? Is this truly a priority? Do you know the effort and sacrifice that it will entail? Oftentimes we have grand visions of epic change because we're in a highly motivated state. New Year's resolutions are a perfect example of this. One of the common traits that exist within resolutions is that they're often wildly unsustainable. The reason for this is simple. Over the holidays, many people eat more freely, drink more alcohol, and typically don't feel very good about their overall health and nutrition. As humans, we are frequently enticed by the concept of a fresh start. We have that New Year celebration as the last chance to live it up before we get our stuff together. It puts us in a highly motivated state to make a change and "undo the damage." However, a small and sustainable goal doesn't excite us enough. We need a bold, ambitious goal. Often it includes many fundamental behavior changes that will require a lot of sacrifice and discipline. Simply put, we routinely bite off more than we can chew each year. That's why most resolutions fail relatively quickly. The mood that you were in when you pronounced this epic change that was going to happen is not the mood you'll be in when the work starts. You may stay motivated initially but like any emotion, it will come and go. What happens when you're no longer motivated? That's why it's important to connect to the deeper meaning as to why this change is important to you. This is why it's also important to start with something that's realistic and achievable. Using 1-2 small goals may not be exciting but is a highly effective way to build confidence in your ability to execute. Then, we can add layers on top of the foundation that we're building. Once you've decided that you're ready for change, you know why it matters to you, and you set realistic goals, the next step is to plan for setbacks.

What obstacles are going to come up? What are the barriers? What are the challenges that are preventing you from changing? Can you assess why you haven't made this change already? What have you already experienced in the past that has prevented you from making that change already? Then, we can anticipate some of those barriers. We have to expect failure to occur. There is no way around it, only through it. It can help accept this as a part of the process by reframing what failure means. There was a cool study that just came out that showed that failure is actually a prerequisite for success. We simply have to look at these setbacks differently. We want to expect them to happen because it is literally a prerequisite for you to be successful. So what relapses can we anticipate happening? What are some of those failures that we can envision? Do you have any triggers that might return you to a previous behavior? Maybe you were already on your weight loss journey in the past and you were doing well, but something triggered you to default back to your previous habits. Maybe it was an argument or maybe it was a traumatic experience. Maybe it was something that happened in your life or in your career that caused you to relapse and caused you to default back to your previous behaviors. Once we analyze those things, then we can best move forward. There is a stage of change model that was made famous in the late 1970s from researchers who were studying ways to help people quit smoking. The stages of change model gained more popularity and have been very effective at helping people understand how to go through any change in behavior. It states that the way we should approach behavior change is gradual with failures as an inevitable part of the process.

We're looking at life-long changes. We're not looking at a quick fix. I want to be very upfront and mention if your goal is to accomplish something as fast as humanly possible, then this book is definitely not for you. If you are looking for a lifelong solution, then you will definitely want to keep reading. Let's look at the approach to changing your behavior. The methods will look different for everyone but the principles will remain the same.

Stage one of the process is the precontemplation stage. In that stage, you're not even considering a change. You're often in denial and likely unaware that your behavior is even a problem. Some of the characteristics are that you might be ignoring a problem that's right in front of you. You might have a fixed mindset. You might be in denial that change needs to happen. Some strategies to help are journaling, being more introspective and self-analytical, creating more self-awareness, rethinking some of your behaviors, assessing what you're currently doing. Consider if what you're doing is serving you and whether you're at a place that you want to be. Ask yourself some questions. What do you feel like your problems are? What do you feel like some of the barriers are going to be if you do attempt to change this behavior?

At *stage two*, we move into the contemplation stage which is more ambivalence and potentially some conflicting emotions. Some days you feel like yes, I definitely want to do this. Other days, you'll think, I'm not really sure if this is for me. This stage can last a very long time. There's a lot of people who never make it past the contemplation stage. You might view change as something that is a massive challenge and something that you just don't want to tackle. Some ways to manage that are by actually writing out the pros and cons of that behavior change. Then consider if you're actually ready and able to create this change and continue to identify some of the barriers that might arise.

Once you determine that this is something you want to change, in this example, prioritizing your health and fitness. Then you move into *stage three*, which is preparation. You may have already started making some smaller changes in your life. You might have started to pay more attention to the types of foods that you're eating or you might have already started scouting a gym. You're experimenting at this point, you're collecting more information, you're reading about different diets. You're in this information gathering stage of preparation, and now you can write down what your actual goals are. It helps to be specific because a lot of people start off too fast. They go from the preparation stage to making a bunch of changes all at once, which just sets them up for failure. Write down your specific goals and then create an action plan to accomplish them. We also want to utilize some of the strategies to create more of a growth mindset. Journal and practice gratitude. Draw off of past experiences and remember a time where you were able to create lasting change in your life. This is all about improving your readiness for change and entering the right frame of mind.

Start to assess how you can make the process easier on yourself. Maybe it's scheduling out some time to get to the gym. Or maybe it's doing some grocery shopping and meal prep to simplify your nutrition plan.

Stage four would be the action stage where you're taking direct action from the plan that you set out to accomplish your goals. During the action stage, we want to set up a reward system for some of the actions that we are taking. For example, if I go to the gym three days this week, I'm going to treat myself to a massage. You can start seeking out social support by having an accountability partner or fitness community. We can even tie an action to the habit we're trying to create. For example, I'm going to meet my friend at the gym to work out together, or I'm going to text my friend after I finish each workout. These are ways that we can enhance the likelihood of following through on an action. It's also important that we don't solely rely on external rewards and motivation. We have to be internally driven, which goes back to having a deep connection with why this even matters in the first place. Because we have to understand that failure is a part of the process and a prerequisite for success. We have to operate with grace and forgiveness for ourselves.

As we go through this action phase we want to constantly reassess what we're doing. Is it moving you forward and do you enjoy the process? Reassess your belief in yourself through that process. Oftentimes, some of those fixed mindset thoughts pop back up and we want to constantly check in with ourselves to catch them before they become too ingrained. This can be accomplished through journaling, through a check-in call with a coach, through having an accountability partner, etc. We want to have systems in place where you'll be able to catch yourself with some of those self-limiting beliefs that are preventing you from moving forward. As we periodically review what you're doing, we want to keep the proper mindset in place because we know that challenging times are going to happen. You're not always going to be motivated. You're not always going to be excited by the process, however, you're going to be disciplined because you understand the benefits of following through is much greater than the detriments of giving up.

As we move through the action phase, we end up in the maintenance phase, which is where most diet programs fall short. When we look at behavior change, a lot of people can force themselves to follow through on a diet, even if they don't enjoy it. We have some people who have the ability to just follow through no matter what. They're rule followers and they want to be compliant, which is just human nature. They set out a goal, for example, maybe it's a 30-day challenge or a six-week challenge, and they decide I'm going to stick this out no matter what. What typically happens is they fail at the maintenance phase. They fall back into their previous habits because they weren't actually learning sustainable practices. They were just following rules that were set for them. They weren't actually following through on something that they wanted for themselves or that was sustainable for them. During that maintenance phase, we really have to reinforce these behaviors. This is where we want those healthy habits to stick. We want to develop certain strategies for resisting falling back into previous behaviors. Something as simple as rearranging your kitchen to stock your fridge with more healthy foods and removing some of the processed foods from your cabinets. Through repetition and time, these habits will become second nature. We've started to form new behaviors, but now we want them to become a part of us. We want it to become like brushing our teeth. We don't have to think much about it, we don't need to be motivated, we just do it.

Once we can get our healthy habits to the point where it's like brushing teeth, then we've won. Now all of a sudden, that is a behavior that will stick for the rest of your life. Then, we can layer on more positive actions. One of the biggest mistakes that people make is that when they're trying to eliminate a bad habit, they often try to white knuckle their way through it. For example, if someone wants to stop eating candy, they often just declare that they want to stop eating candy. They don't do anything fundamentally different. One of the best ways to remove a bad habit is to first replace it with a positive habit. The analogy that I like to give is getting soap out of a soap bottle. The most effective way to do it isn't just by shaking the soap out of the bottle. The best way to do it is to fill it with water. Initially, there's going to be a little bit of water and a little bit of soap. As you continue to fill the bottle with water, now all of a sudden, all the soap has been completely removed from the bottle, and now it's filled with water. Not only did you remove a bad habit, but you've also replaced it with a positive habit.

If you want to clean up your diet, one of the first things to do is add to your diet. Eat more vegetables, drink more water, and eat more lean protein. Add first, which is the equivalent of adding water to the soap bottle. Adding more naturally will allow you to remove that bad habit more effectively. You'll get to the point where you don't even want to do that bad habit anymore because it doesn't align with your goals and doesn't like how it makes you feel. You might start to notice that because you're eating more vegetables because you're drinking more water, that all a sudden you don't crave candy as much. And when you do eat candy, it gives you an energy crash and you feel like crap. Now you have an intrinsic desire to continue to pursue behaviors and actions that make you feel better.

One effective strategy is that we want to stack positive habits on top of other habits that already exist. The more specific that we can get with habit creation, the more likely it is to sustain. An example of this would be, let's say that every single morning at 8 am you drink coffee. Well, if I wanted to add a 10-minute walk to my day, one thing I could do is stack that habit so every single morning at 8:10 am after I drink my morning coffee, I'm going to go for a 10-minute walk.

The existing habit is the cue or trigger for the habit I want to acquire. Specificity is extremely important. I'm going to give an example from least effective to most effective. The least effective would be, I want to walk more. A little bit better than that would be, I want to walk for 10 minutes a day. A little bit better than that would be I want to walk for 10 minutes a day, five days a week. A little bit better than that would be I want to walk for 10 minutes a day, five days a week, Monday through Friday. A little bit better than that would be I want to walk for 10 minutes a day, five days a week, Monday through Friday at 8:10 am. And even better than that would be I want to walk 10 minutes a day, five days a week, Monday through Friday at 8:10 am after I drink my coffee. That's going to be the most effective because it's super-specific. The existing habit triggers the new task and the more we can do that, the more likely we're going to be able to maintain that habit.

We also have to look at removing the friction for a positive habit and increasing the friction for a negative habit. When we talk about friction, it's simply making a negative habit more difficult to accomplish. If I have candy readily accessible at all times of the day, at my work desk, on the counter in my kitchen, there's not a lot of friction between me and the candy. Now if I hide the candy or place it in a high cabinet and put it away, there's a lot of friction between me and the candy. There was an interesting study that showed just how powerful friction can be in eliciting a more positive outcome. This was done at an office building where every employee took the elevator instead of the stairs. The researchers programmed a slight delay in the elevator so it wouldn't be as easily accessible. The delayed response time on the elevator caused the employees to take the stairs to their office. Similarly, with the positive habit, we want to decrease the amount of friction. Let's say that I want to go for a walk at 8:10 am after I drink my coffee every morning. Some ways to decrease the friction would be to have my walking shoes by the door and have my coat ready if it's a cold day. Place everything out in visible sight so when I come downstairs in the morning, it's right there. There's not a lot of effort required. It's simply going out and doing it. We can even attach it to another positive habit like perhaps I want to listen to 10 minutes of an audio book while I take my walk. Now there's an even greater incentive. It's like rewarding yourself for accomplishing that task. I get to listen to a book that I really want to listen to and I'm going to do it while I'm taking my morning walk. We've stacked these positive changes on top of each other.

Throughout the maintenance phase, we've gone through this process, we've created some change, and we figured out what works best for ourselves. We've got these behaviors that are pretty well established. However, there's going to be a relapse stage. This will typically conjure up feelings of frustration, feeling like a failure, and feeling disappointed in yourself. First, just start with awareness and the understanding that anytime you create a behavior change, relapses are going to happen. When you go through a relapse, you're going to feel disappointed, you're going to feel like you don't have the ability to be successful.

However, we have to understand that setbacks and failures do not define you. We cannot let them impact self-confidence. The belief that we can create change still exists. At this point, we want to become analytical. We're figuring out this piece of the puzzle. Why did that happen? What can I do to avoid that in the future? Typically, when relapses happen, we can trace back some common trends and understand why it occurred. Even if it's something as simple as the environment that it happened in, like every time I binge eat, I binge eat in the kitchen. Well, now, I can change that environment so when I have this feeling of binge eating, I can go outside. I can remove myself from the environment it happens in. That doesn't guarantee that I won't go back in and binge eat but I've eliminated a common thread for that relapse. If nothing else, it places a pause between my knee-jerk reaction and making a conscious decision. Any time we can take a step back, put ourselves in the present moment, and proceed with a conscious choice we are much more likely to make a positive decision. Assess the situation if it does occur. What are the facts of the situation? Where did it happen? What was I going through? What were the emotions I was feeling? I've had clients who have figured out that their binge eating happened every single time they argued with their spouse. We've been able to develop more productive outlets and coping mechanisms for that argument and we replaced the negative habit with a positive one. The best solution is to assess why it happened, see if there are any common themes, and then start again with better preparation. Go back through the action stage, the maintenance stage, and now we have more tools at our disposal and we're more prepared for the possible setbacks that are going to arise. With the understanding that it may continue to happen, but it'll be fewer and further in between. It's not an easy process to make a change, but it's so worth it. When you have an understanding of how behavior change takes place, it becomes a much more effortless process, even though it still takes work.

One last note, when we rely solely on discipline and willpower, we're really setting ourselves up for failure. Assess the changes that you're trying to make and consider if you are tapping into your discipline and willpower too much. Think of willpower as a finite resource or like a battery that can get charged or drained. Just like the battery on your phone, you wouldn't leave it unplugged all day long and then expect it to work properly in a couple of days. It's the same thing when you rely solely on willpower. If you are putting yourself in a position where you have to walk by junk food all day, you're draining that willpower battery. You have to establish a way to recharge, and ideally, remove the thing that is draining your battery. We can't rely solely on discipline and willpower, although they will be required in small doses, we want to save them for when we need them the most. That's an important thing to understand. Take inventory of whether you're operating with a high dependence on discipline and willpower. Think about that in terms of the dietary practices that you're doing. If you're eliminating entire food groups or labeling foods as good versus bad food, you're tapping into that willpower battery and it's only a matter of time until you break. The process of habit creation and behavior change includes setting up your environment for success.

CHAPTER 7

NEUROPLASTICITY: THE SECRET SCIENCE-BASED
APPROACH TO REWIRING YOUR BRAIN

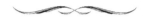

Do you ever have that feeling where you're not sure if you're awake or still dreaming? This quote is from the famous Hollywood movie, "The Matrix." The Matrix does a great job of capturing this concept that our perception becomes our reality. The Matrix is all around us proclaims Morpheus to Neo as he just awakes. Now, the symbolic reference made in The Matrix is interesting because it opened up this concept that's been around for quite some time that the world is basically a super-imposition on our minds. It's like a mirage that our dream state and reality are intertwined and the things that we perceive to be true, actually become our reality. What's interesting is that we typically choose the path of seeking comfort and pleasure, which would be equal to choosing the blue pill from The Matrix. Freedom lies not in having a good dream, but in knowing that it's all a dream. An important concept to understand is that questioning the solid reality of our daily life is a good place to start because it helps you step back from all of the fears, doubts, and disbelief and allows you to truly

74

open your mind to what's possible. What's fascinating is the science to support what happens when we change our perceptions and our thoughts, which is known as Neuroplasticity.

Our brains are constantly being shaped by the experiences that we have and the thoughts that enter our mind. The shift in how our brain is shaped is known as Neuroplasticity. Our brain changes structure as we continue to experience things, learn new things and adapt. As humans, we are adaptive by nature. Every single repetition, every single action, every single thought or emotion, we reinforce this neurological pathway, or neurons firing down a certain path. If you think about it like riding your bike through a dirt path, the first time that you take that path, you're not going to leave much of a trail. However, if you ride that same path, thousands of times over again, there's going to be quite a divot made in the dirt. That is similar to having these pre-existing beliefs that we repeat over and over to ourselves. That is similar to having a fixed mindset. I can give a personal example of this. When I was in high school, I had an English teacher who read one of my papers and bluntly stated that I just wasn't a good writer. Now, the first time that I heard that, it was like the first time I rode my bike through that path, it didn't really leave much of a trail. As I continued throughout my life, it stuck with me. The more that I repeated that thought in my brain, the more that path became ingrained in me. It became my reality. My perception of my ability to perform as a writer became my reality and that neural pathway became ingrained in my brain.

It wasn't until I challenged that self-limiting belief when I was asked to do an assignment for a company I was working for. It was a writing assignment and all of a sudden, I was struck with anxiety as I sat down to write because I kept telling myself that I'm not a good writer. What occurred to me was that the self-limiting belief was not even my own. It was imposed upon me and then I reinforced it by repeating that story over and over in my head. I realized that it became a self-fulfilling prophecy because by telling myself I'm not a good writer, I never actually wrote anything. And the only way to get better is through repetition and practice. At that point, I wrote the assignment and began writing as a daily habit.

The cool thing about Neuroplasticity is that by breaking that existing thought pattern, my brain actually changed its shape. There's a new pathway for neurons to travel so that old path that I rode my bike on faded away, and there was a new path that was created. That is the concept of Neuroplasticity. It's like muscle building for the brain. The things that we do frequently, we become stronger at, and the things that we don't use fade away. That's why it's important to understand that having a thought or an action, repeated over and over again, increases its power. If we look at it from a health perspective, we want to get to the point of creating healthy habits that become automatic. They become a part of us and our brain literally develops these ingrained pathways that neurons will travel down, allowing us to accomplish what we're trying to accomplish. Getting to the point where we don't even have to think about it. We literally become the version of what we think and repeatedly do.

Neuroplasticity can occur all throughout life. Different connections within the brain are constantly strengthening or weakening and that really opens up the ability to foster a growth mindset. There's so much that we can do to mold who we are and what we're capable of if we just harness the power of Neuroplasticity. This can be applied to improving our fitness and becoming a healthier version of ourselves. It can be applied in trying to advance in our careers, improve relationships, get better at communication, and all the things that will lead to a better life.

The interesting thing about Neuroplasticity is the impact that exercise has on our brain chemistry. In the 1990s, researchers discovered something that challenged a relatively standard belief in the world of neuroscience. For decades, scientists believed that the mature brain was incapable of growing new neurons. Many studies have since emerged showing that something as simple as exercising, can lead to the birth of new neurons. Current literature even suggests that exercise, especially as we age, may help reduce the risk of Alzheimer's disease and other neurodegenerative conditions.

Research is showing that exercise actually increases the sensitivity of the reward and pleasure centers of our brain. Dopamine is the neurotransmitter that's responsible for that pleasure-seeking or that reward response in the brain and it's actually the dopaminergic system that we have to look at when it comes to how we respond to things that are joyful. Simply having dopamine present doesn't necessarily guarantee that there's going to be a pleasure response because it has to do with the system as a whole. The receptors for dopamine have to be sensitive to the dopamine that you're producing and exercise actually improves dopamine sensitivity, so it improves the sensitivity of the dopaminergic receptors.

In other words, when we engage in a consistent exercise routine, life, in general, becomes more pleasurable. We enjoy things more and what an amazing concept, to be able to use a healthy habit like exercise to actually improve quality of life outside of just the physical benefits. There's no doubt about the physical benefits when it comes to exercise but to be able to literally improve how you enjoy life, and how you perceive different experiences just through exercise, is an amazing thing. Combine that with the impact that it has on molding your brain and increasing the sensitivity and the effectiveness of the dopaminergic system, and it's really a practice that everyone should have. As if we needed more reasons to exercise, current literature shows that exercise plays on the endocannabinoid system, which will improve contentment and sense of well being. In addition, we'll see an endorphin release and other chemical messengers throughout the body, that just through exercise, we're increasing these hormones, these neurotransmitters, and their effects on the body.

We also know that on the flip side of that, exercise is a powerful antidepressant. Not only are we enjoying life more by exercising because we're increasing the effectiveness of the reward center of the brain, but we're also, on the other side, decreasing the likelihood of becoming depressed. Even for medical and therapeutic methods of dealing with depression, exercise on top of that will increase the effectiveness of the medication and therapy. There's literally nothing else to my knowledge at this time that has that kind of an impact on your brain chemistry.

It stands to reason that one of the most powerful healthy habits that we can consistently do is take part in a steady exercise routine. It is something that we see in people who are successful within their fitness journey. We know that by repetitively doing this habit over and over again, it's going to, through Neuroplasticity, ingrain that neural pathway to make that a part of us. It becomes who we are. We identify as somebody who exercises. Using your identity is another effective strategy for habit creation. Rather than saying, I want to exercise, it's better to identify as the person who already does this. It's more advantageous to say, I am someone who exercises, and now by identifying as that person, your actions will align with who you want to be. Then the more repetitions that you put in, the more ingrained it will become in your daily life.

Another part of Neuroplasticity is the impact that something like gratitude has on your brain chemistry. There were Psychologists from the University of California and the University of Miami, who published a study in 2015 that looked at the physical outcomes of practicing gratitude. They had a third of their subjects keep a daily journal of things that happened throughout the week for which they were grateful. Another third, they were asked to write down the daily irritations of their week. And then they had the last group that was asked to write down situations that really had no effect one way or the other on their emotional stability. So it was just kind of an event that happened that was neutral. At the end of the 10-week study, each group was asked to record how they felt physically and generally about life. The gratitude group reported feeling more optimistic and positive about their lives than the two other groups. Also, the gratitude group was more physically active and reported fewer visits to the doctor than those who only wrote about their negative experiences. So not just from overall enjoyment, but from actual physical health, a simple practice like gratitude can have a profound effect.

Other researchers have studied the physical results by looking at brain chemistry a little bit more closely. They wanted to focus on the effects of how positive thinking and feeling grateful can improve your sleep quality and reduce your feelings of anxiety and depression. They also found that levels of gratitude correlated with better mood, less fatigue, less inflammation and also reduced the risk of heart failure, even for those who are already susceptible to heart failure. There was an experiment conducted at the University of California where brain activity was measured using magnetic resonance imaging. They asked subjects a question and induced them to feel gratitude by giving them a gift. The areas of the brain showing increased activity were the anterior cortex and the medial prefrontal cortex, which were associated with moral and social cognition, reward, empathy and value judgment, leading them to the conclusion that the emotion of gratitude supports a positive and supportive attitude towards others, and a feeling of relief towards stressors. Gratitude activates the hypothalamus as well and that has downstream effects on the metabolism, stress and other various behaviors. From a health standpoint, a mindfulness practice such as daily gratitude can have major benefits. It can improve your emotional health, physical health, metabolism, and can even impact things like hunger, appetite, and sleep quality. The positive influence on mental health is something that is continuously studied, and consistently shows the positive impacts that gratitude has on mental health. Something simple like keeping a daily journal for the things that you're grateful for is a great habit. Make it a point to tell the people in your life that you appreciate them. Even when you look at yourself in the mirror each morning, take a moment to tell yourself out loud, something that you're proud of, something that you're appreciative of, or something that you like about yourself. A daily affirmation in the morning can have a massive impact on your health. And as we know, repeating those acts will mold your brain and it will become a part of who you are.

The understanding of neuroplasticity really fosters more of a growth mindset. It allows you to focus on healthy habit formation, and it can help your perceptions become your reality. If your perceptions are more positive, encouraging, and empowering, you're going to be more successful in the long-term. Many people view their health journey with a start and end date but we want to change that perspective. We must understand that this is something you need to do for the rest of your life. By understanding neuroplasticity, and using different tools like an exercise routine and a daily mindfulness practice, we can stack the deck in our favor for sustaining long term results.

CHAPTER 8

FOOD AND MOOD

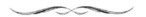

One of the first diets that I ever went on, I received a grocery list that had a good foods column and a bad foods column. I went into this diet program very excited and highly motivated to make a change. I went to the grocery store so I could pick out all of my "good" foods to stock my kitchen. I remember wanting to grab some apples and carrots, two foods that I enjoy quite a bit. Trying to incorporate more fruits and vegetables I thought was a good idea. Then I looked down at my bad list and realized that staring me right in the face was both apples and carrots. The reasoning for those foods being on the bad list, I am still unclear. I did go back to the person that gave me the list and asked why, out of curiosity, am I not allowed to eat apples and carrots, and the response that I got was, just follow the plan. So I did. I stayed on that diet for a while and ended up getting to a very low weight that I had not seen in a long time. To put things in perspective, my original goal when I was 250 pounds was that I just wanted to get below 200 pounds. When I went on this diet, I was probably around 210 pounds, and I quickly got below 200 but that wasn't good enough. So I thought maybe I just need to get below 190. At that point, I kept sticking very religiously to my good foods list and I got below 190 and that still didn't feel good enough. So I thought, you know what, I just need to be below 180 in order for me to feel good. I had some moments of wanting to quit, I had some moments of feeling restricted by the limited list of foods that were acceptable, but I kept pushing through. Finally, I got below 180 and that still didn't feel right. I would look at myself in the mirror and I was not satisfied with the way I looked. I didn't like anything about myself at that time. I was still riddled with insecurities and I still didn't have the confidence that I thought these arbitrary weight goals would give me so I just kept going. Eventually, I got down into the 160s. And at that point, I remember feeling like I just needed a break to not feel like a prisoner to my diet. Well, that ended in an epic binge, where, if I remember correctly, I ate 12 slices of pizza and somewhere in the neighborhood of 10 cookies within about an hour. That led me down the path of constantly restricting and bingeing and yo-yo dieting in the traditional sense.

What I didn't realize was that by following this food list and labeling foods as good versus bad, that I was tarnishing and destroying my relationship with food and my relationship with my body. We often only think of food in terms of nourishment, in terms of energy, in terms of providing some sort of a caloric load and we don't realize that food is so much more than that. Food is emotional, food is social, food can be used for celebration, food can be used to connect with people. It can be something to stir up memories, it can be something that brings families together. So to have tunnel vision when it comes to food and only think about it in terms of energy is really ignoring all of the other aspects that it provides when we're talking about food and overall well being.

I learned the hard way. "Have you heard of orthorexia?" I squirmed in my chair. I can remember the exact restaurant and the exact chair that I was sitting in when those words were uttered to me. They were not the words of a stranger or even just an acquaintance. They were the words of someone very close to me. "Orthorexia is disordered eating where there's an obsession over 'healthy' or 'clean' foods, she said. I got incredibly defensive. Even though several minutes earlier I had just ordered a salad with grilled chicken breast and emphatically expressed that I did not want them using any oil or butter when cooking. I also told the server to hold the cheese, croutons, and dressing. You mean, dressing on the side, she asked? No. I mean no dressing at all. The good vs bad food list that I received triggered my perfectionist tendencies and I refused to stay from the plan. I swore it was in the name of just wanting to be healthy. I guess I confused health with being anti-social and having crippling anxiety being around foods that aren't allowed. It's possible I confused health with being the smallest version of myself and still not satisfied, happy, or fulfilled. Anyway, I snapped back at the comments about orthorexia. You know those moments where you get so defensive about something and you realize later on there was a reason for it? That's because it struck a chord. Her words hit me in the gut and I could feel it. I ignored that feeling for quite some time. The psychological damage of this mindset coupled with the restriction and binge habit forced me to make a change. I

84

had to find my way out. I had to develop a better relationship with food and my body. It was a long and arduous road but necessary and worth it.

Your relationship with food is going to be so important for long term success when it comes to your health. Having a healthy relationship with food means not labeling foods as good versus bad, but understanding the foods that make you feel your best, the foods that nourish you, and understanding the context of when certain foods make you feel better than others. In other words, you might have certain foods that fuel your workout better than others and you might have certain foods that fuel your relationships better than others. In the context of wanting to be with your family and connecting over a good meal, you might choose a slice of pizza and a glass of wine, even though it's not providing value to the physical side of your health. It's improving your relationship with your family, it's improving the social, the familial side, probably the emotional and maybe even the spiritual side of your health. We have to look at the big picture and understand health as this all-encompassing sphere and not be so narrow-focused when it comes to food. However, there are certain foods that are engineered to drive us to overeat. We don't want to label these foods as bad, however, we do want to create an awareness around these foods and be mindful of how we incorporate them into our lives. Highly processed foods might be best utilized only on rare occasions because we know they don't serve much in terms of nutrient value and there is a lot of processing and engineering that goes into making these foods that will cause us to overeat and will alter the chemical makeup of our brains. Food has a profound impact on neurotransmitter balance. Neurotransmitters are simply chemical messengers that circulate throughout the body and send signals that impact our emotions, our actions, how we feel. Basically, everything that we do is driven by some sort of neurotransmitter, chemical reaction. And foods will impact the neurotransmitter balance in your body. Here's one example of how processed foods can make us feel worse. There is a neurotransmitter called glutamate, which is almost like our emotional amplifier. It also plays a role in memory but glutamate is something that enhances the emotional response to something. And there are fast food companies who have placed glutamate into their food to make the emotional response and the addictive properties of that food higher.

Imagine eating a fast-food burger and it's triggering the pleasure center of your brain, but it's also increasing the emotional response. Now, consider how badly you'll want to eat that burger again and how much you'd want to eat more of it. It's overriding your natural signals of satiety and causing you to consume more than you normally would, if it were just simply an unprocessed, whole food. Therefore, we want to create awareness around certain foods without the labels of good versus bad or thinking "I can eat this but I can't eat that." There was a study that was done by Kevin Hall to investigate the impact of highly processed foods versus an unprocessed diet and they had 20 adults who received an ultra-processed diet versus an unprocessed diet for 14 days each and then they switched. The diets were matched for calories, sugar, fat, fiber and macronutrients. And then there was a period of ad-libitum intake. And the ultra-processed diet resulted in 500 calories per day more than the unprocessed diet and the bodyweight changes were highly correlated with the dietary differences in energy intake. In other words, the subjects who ate more during the ultra-processed diet phase would gain weight because they were over-consuming calories. This is due to the nature of highly processed foods and having food engineers whose literal job is to get you to over-consume that food. They want you to eat more of it because then you have to buy more of it. And this is a multi-billion dollar industry in it of itself. Food engineers go through many different variations to come up with the perfect profile of taste, salt, fat and even consider the texture and things like the crunch of a chip, which will cause overconsumption. In addition to that, neurotransmitters are involved and we have something like glutamate that's added to foods and it's also playing on our dopamine receptors and increasing the pleasure response we obtain from that food. Well, now we're really going to go out of our way to consume that food.

There is also an association between different high processed foods and certain experiences. That's why when you go to a movie theater, without even thinking about it, your natural instinct is to grab a bag of popcorn with a lot of butter and a soft drink. This is something that was created to play to the habitual nature of humans. We understand that going through the motions and mindless eating, it interrupts our natural signals of satiety. You'll see bags of popcorn that are way oversized and bigger than anything you would buy in the store or make at home. First of all, they're hijacking our natural signals of satiety. Secondly, they're playing on this mindless eating behavior of being distracted while we eat which makes it much easier to overconsume. What we want to do is simply create awareness around some of these behaviors and habits. We don't want to label these foods as bad or say we can't eat them. Having rules like that around food is well documented as being highly ineffective. We want to understand the impact that food has on us and why we're prone to overeat these foods.

Often there are feelings of guilt and shame associated with eating something that might be "bad" for you. Now, we don't want to feel guilty or shameful about it because we have very strong evidence that supports the fact that if you feel guilty or shameful about your body weight or your eating behaviors, you're actually less likely to make a change. In other words, feeling bad about yourself might drive you to make an initial change. But the statistics are clear that it is a very poor indicator for long term change. A better and more sustainable approach is that you're making these decisions because you're coming from a place of self-love and self-respect. You have awareness around how these foods are engineered and how they make you feel. This puts the control back in your hands and empowers you to make decisions that align with your goals. We have to understand that it's nothing to be ashamed of because we're dealing with experts in their craft. If you were to race Usain Bolt, you wouldn't beat yourself up over losing the race, you're racing one of the fastest humans on the earth, you understand the deck is stacked against you. And it's the same thing when you over-consume processed foods. There are food engineers, who are much smarter than we are and their sole job is to make foods hyper-palatable and highly seductive. You're playing against an expert, and it really is nothing to feel bad about. Once we understand that, it's much easier to make decisions based on our own personal preferences and goals.

Then we can assess different situations and make the choices that fit within the context of our lifestyle. Using the family example, if I want to get together with my family and enjoy a slice of pizza, I understand the place that it has in my life and the part of my health that it's serving. I no longer have to feel guilty about that choice. Understanding the impact that food has on mood through the disruption or the support of neurotransmitters can be very enlightening. There is a lot we can do, simply from a food quality standpoint. We know that dopamine is the pleasure center or the reward center of the brain, foods that are high in protein, specifically the amino acid l-tyrosine will support dopamine production. Foods that are high in choline, like eggs, will support acetylcholine production which is a neurotransmitter that's responsible for motor learning, memory, and coordination. Foods that are high in l-taurine, which is another amino acid, will support the production of GABA, which is the neurotransmitter that calms our brain down. So it helps us fight against anxiety and fear. Foods that are high in l-Tryptophan, like certain proteins and carbohydrates, will support the production of serotonin, which will provide feelings of contentment and well-being.

Now, we look at the quality of these foods, we want to look at mostly whole, natural foods. The ultimate goal here is to create awareness. Understanding and looking at foods in the specific context of what part of your health are they supporting at that time, and then making conscious decisions to coincide with that.

CHAPTER 9

NUTRITION IDEOLOGY

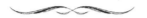

There were a couple of famous studies done at Stanford University to assess why humans seem to not change their beliefs in the face of facts. Essentially, what they did was they put students through various tests, and they were actually being deceived throughout the entire study but they would come up with a conclusion before they were told that all the facts were not true. The students would read these different notes and they would come up with a conclusion based on the notes. At the end of the study, they were told that none of the notes were actually true. But what the observers found was that once their conclusions were formed, despite showing evidence to the contrary, their conclusions were remarkably difficult to dissuade. They were very firm in their beliefs. There was a follow-up study that was also done at Stanford, basically showing the same thing.

The students were asked to describe their own beliefs about a firefighter and what sort of attitude towards risk they believe that a successful firefighter would have. They were given a packet beforehand that would kind of guide them to their answer. So, one of the packets indicated that a successful firefighter would avoid risk and another packet was given that indicated that a successful firefighter would embrace risk. Even after the evidence, which for their beliefs had been totally refuted, the students would fail to make the appropriate revisions in their beliefs. The conductors of the study were quoted as saying that it was particularly impressive how steadfast they were in their beliefs, that was refuted directly after the conclusion had been revealed. And it begs the question as to why it's so challenging for us to change pre-existing beliefs. There have been several theories as to why this is, one of which talks about it from an evolutionary standpoint, because humans survived and thrived largely due to our ability to cooperate and exist in groups.

We often see various groups being formed and that has led to a concept known as confirmation bias. Simply put, confirmation bias is that whenever I believe something, I will go out of my way to find all of the facts that support my existing beliefs, and everybody else who has similar beliefs. We feel a part of a community and that feeling of camaraderie and that feeling of belonging has helped us survive as a species for as long as we have. So, whenever there is something that flies in the face of your beliefs, we typically are very stubborn and often avoid being open minded. We avoid seeing things from another perspective because it threatens the group that we're a part of and it threatens that camaraderie. We use those groups as support systems and that's why we see things that are so divisive like politics, like religion, and unfortunately, like nutrition. Nutrition ideology is something that has caused a lot of confusion in space because

91

there are different groups out there who want you to believe that there is one best way to approach your nutrition. We see examples of this all over the place but some popular ones that we have are proponents of a vegan diet. You have people who have almost created a cult-like atmosphere in support of a vegan diet, and they want you to believe that it is the best way to eat. The fact is, there is nothing wrong with wanting to eat a vegan diet, the issue is when it's being represented as the best diet for everyone and any disagreement is met with a personal attack.

On the extreme other end, there is something known as the carnivore diet in which you're eating, no plants and only animal products, mostly red meat. Carnivore advocates want you to believe that plants are causing more harm than they are doing good and that vegans are misinformed and that everybody should be eating this way. We also see a diet like the ketogenic diet, which has regained popularity. The ketogenic diet is simply very low in carbohydrates, moderate to low protein and very high in fat and there are a lot of keto advocates who believe that this is the most effective way to lose weight. You also have those on the high carb side who feel like fats are worse for your health so they should be kept lower, and that carbs should be kept higher. You see this battle going back and forth between groups with opposing views. It's almost to the point where nutrition becomes like a religion, people are identifying very strongly with their dietary choices and that leads to a very confused consumer. Because you can have two people on opposing sides of the spectrum, who are both quoting different parts of research using confirmation bias, cherry-picking data that suits their argument and you can end up as a very lost consumer trying to find the best approach for you.

The important thing to understand through all of this is that there is no one size fits all approach to dieting, that nutrition is not an either-or type of deal. It's possible that you can try different things, experiment, and see what works best for you. The bottom line is that we are all individuals with individual needs. So even though Keto might be the best approach for somebody else, and maybe it's somebody that's very close to you, that doesn't mean that it's going to work well for you. When we look at the best way to approach certain nutritional ideologies, is to start to test and see how that fits through your own personal lens. If you do have somebody who wants you to try a vegan diet, rather than trying to argue with them about why it might not be the best fit, think about it through your own personal lens. How would that fit within your lifestyle? How easy would it be to follow? Would it be sustainable? And does it allow you to do the things in your life that are meaningful for you? Let's use the example of a ketogenic diet, where you're basically eliminating all carbohydrates, is that really something that you could adhere to or sustain for the rest of your life? And if it is, then that might be a solid approach for you. If you are someone who enjoys carbs, whether it be due to personal preference or because of your training style, or just because you would find it very restrictive to cut out an entire food group, well then keto is probably not the best approach.

Rather than trying to find this one size fits all nutrition plan, we want to be like metabolic detectives and nutritional detectives in finding what fits best for us. How something makes you feel, how it allows you to perform, how easy it is to adhere to, how it fits within your lifestyle and does it allow you to enjoy the things that are meaningful in your life. If you're somebody that likes to travel, your dietary choices or your nutrition plan should accommodate and allow for you to travel without having to stress whether or not you're able to stay consistent. If you are somebody who likes to be social and you like to have a drink or two on the weekends, your nutrition plan should allow for that level of flexibility. And if you find yourself having to remove things in your life that are very enjoyable, just for the sake of staying consistent with your nutrition, you're sacrificing a big part of your health, outside of just physical. We always have to remember the psychological impact that dieting can have. I remember many nights that I would cancel on friends or I wouldn't go out to see my family because I knew that trying to be social didn't fit within the very restrictive diet plan that I was on. I missed out on a lot of experiences and memories that I can't get back. When we assess a nutrition protocol, rather than getting married to the idea of one size fits all, let's truly look at it from a personal standpoint. And if we can, it helps not to project our own beliefs onto other people, even though we understand that we like to be a part of a group and we like to feel like we belong. It's possible to have a strong support system or be a part of a community where the common goal is better health. Where each person is on their own individual path and the community celebrates that individuality while supporting each other.

94

When it comes to nutrition, we can truly all be on the same page for better health. We can zoom out and look at the fact that if we're all healthier, even if that means that one person's doing vegan and the other person is doing carnivore if that makes us all healthier, then we all win and we're all part of the same community anyway, so we really don't have to have these arguments. It's like we're having the wrong conversations over and over again, trying to show off about different studies and facts about certain dietary choices. Most of the time they don't apply to the individual who's reading it or hearing it.

Even when we look at certain studies it's important to remember that studies only report the averages. Within each study, individual variance is going to exist across the board. That means that the individual response to certain protocols is going to be different. So looking at things from the lens of your own personal perspective, how things will make you feel, how sustainable it will be is truly the best way to assess. It always comes back to adherence, sustainability, and consistency, and if we can apply those things to ourselves, it will help us find the protocol that works best for us.

The other issue with nutrition ideologies and arguments about which diet is "best," is they often give the appearance that you, as the consumer, have to choose one or the other. A famous example of how this can play out on a massive scale is by looking back at the popular TV commercials for Pepsi and Coke. Remember those "which tastes better" commercials, which I believe started as far back as the 1970s? There would be a blind taste test and the commercial would display people choosing their pick for the better tasting soda. If it was a Pepsi commercial, the results would obviously favor Pepsi. If it was a Coke commercial, the results would favor Coke. The true brilliance of these ads was not that they concluded anything significant about the better tasting soda. The true brilliance was giving the general consumer the impression that they only had two choices when it came to their soda preference! Pepsi and Coke were able to take away all of the market shares from smaller soda brands because the consumer believed there were only two choices. It was presented as an either-or situation. Which is the same thing that happens when we try to argue about our dietary preferences. True nutritional success comes from finding what works best for you, as an individual. Being led to believe you have to choose a pre-established nutrition plan is grossly inaccurate and damaging. The answer lies in all the variables that make you the unique individual that you are. There is no way that a one size fits all diet can solve for that.

CHAPTER 10

NUTRITION FUNDAMENTALS

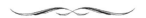

The basics of Nutrition will get you very far in your journey. When you look at every successful transformation, they all have one thing in common, the methodologies and the principles may be different but there is always a consistent execution of the basics for a very long period of time. We all want to believe that there's some shortcut or secret sauce that we're missing, that we just haven't unpacked yet or we haven't discovered yet. The reality is that advanced methods and protocols really serve nothing more than a distraction from what truly matters. If we execute the fundamentals consistently, then we're going to get very far in achieving the health and fitness goals that we want to accomplish. This chapter is going to outline the foundation for everything that you need to know with regards to nutrition. Simply following the fundamentals, you'll be able to get 90% of the way there. It's not flashy, it's not overly exciting, but it is 100% necessary.

Nutritional science is a constantly evolving field and there's a lot of stuff that people don't agree on and we see a lot of conflicting information out there. The fundamentals and the basics have stood the test of time and these are things that we all can agree on. So it stands to reason that we should focus most of our attention on the basics. So, this is like the engine, tires, gas and all the internal workings of your car. And when we get into the advanced methods that's like, what kind of paint do you want to use?

The most important thing above all else is your mindset, which we've been covering throughout this process, but when we talk about nutrition, we have to start with the mindset first because if we look at it simply from the calories in versus calories out discussion, that doesn't help us sustain what we're doing. We're doing a disservice to people if we don't help them understand the importance of mindset first, and allowing the rest to fall into place from there. Most people view their dietary protocol as a temporary solution with a start date and an end date and that's going to yield a temporary result. If you're not in it for the long game, or able to see the big picture, you will fail in the long term. It's the same thing with Training and Fitness. It's the same thing with nutrition. There is a time and a place to get more intentional, for example, if you have an ambitious goal that you want to accomplish. For instance, if you want to compete in bodybuilding. However, for most people, that's going to be unsustainable in the long term. That's part of a greater plan and that's not what I'm referring to. What I'm referring to is just the average person who wants to be fit and healthy, and feel confident and look their best. They don't necessarily even need to have aesthetic goals, but just any form of fitness goal, health goal, etc the basics of nutrition are going to be the catalyst to get you there.

We don't want to view our nutrition as something we're either on or off. We want to view it as something that we do for the rest of our lives. We want to establish these habits and begin to identify as a fit and healthy person, someone who prioritizes themselves, someone who knows that the people around them deserve the best version of themselves. Food is not just fuel, yes, its energy, but it's also emotion. It's social, it's experience, it's pleasure, and we can look at all of the literature on calories in versus calories out until we're blue in the face but we can't ignore the human element when it comes to sustainability and adherence. There's a reason why yo-yo dieting is so prevalent. There's a reason why self-sabotage is so prevalent. There's a reason why a lot of people get tied up into the outcomes of their diet, like solely focusing on a bodyweight goal. There's a reason why a lot of people aren't patient enough to see the results of their hard work. For most people, the reason for all the above is a flawed mindset. You're either still identifying as an unhealthy person and allowing that story to repeat itself in your head, or you're afraid of change, or you're holding on to some ingrained, self-limiting belief. As we've been talking about, fostering more of a growth mindset will allow you to believe that you are in control and that you can create change. It all begins with creating self-awareness, then having the information to execute and taking action on creating that change. Belief in yourself, belief that you want to be the best version of yourself, and understanding that you do, in fact, have control over that. Once we have that mindset in place, now we can get into some of the specifics of nutrition fundamentals. Yes, we do have to look at energy balance, which is simply calories in versus calories out. When we

99

look at calories in, we're talking about the foods and drinks that we consume.

A calorie is just a unit of measurement. It's the energy that we obtain from the foods that we eat. When we look at calories out, we're just looking at the energy that we expend, the energy that we burn on a daily basis. We'll go into the specifics of that in a minute but understand that when it comes to weight gain and weight loss, it is going to be driven by calorie balance. Therefore, if we consume and bring in more calories than we expend, that is going to result in weight gain and if we burn more calories than we consume, that is going to result in weight loss. We want to remember that at the end of the day, it's about being able to sustain what we're doing. Simply creating a calorie deficit and saying that a calorie deficit is all that matters, is really doing us a disservice because it doesn't factor in all of the different individual variables that come into play when we talk about actually adhering to and sustaining that deficit but we do have to understand what that looks like from a scientific standpoint.

When we look at caloric maintenance or the number of calories that you would need just to maintain your current weight, we want to understand what your total daily energy expenditure is. So your total daily energy expenditure or TDEE is going to be comprised of four variables. Your BMR, which is your basal metabolic rate, is essentially how many calories it takes for your body to just keep the lights on. Then we have the thermic effect of food. Actually digesting food requires energy, it requires calories for that process to occur. Then we have non-exercise activity

100

thermogenesis or NEAT, which is every activity or movement outside of the gym, like walking, fidgeting, chores, that sort of thing. And then we have your exercise activity. That is going to be dedicated exercise.

All of these four components will make up your total daily energy expenditure. How many calories you burn on a daily basis is very variable. There are some components that we have more control over than others. The thermic effect of food, we don't have all that much control over. However, we know that protein, as a macronutrient, has the highest thermic effect of food, meaning it requires the most energy to process in the body. So we can increase the number of calories we burn through the digestive process by consuming a higher protein diet, even though the difference would be fairly minimal. We also know that we can't really increase all that much the amount of energy that we burn doing exercise. We could exercise for longer, but eventually, our bodies adapt and we become more efficient. So there's only so much we can do with regards to exercise. Our basal metabolic rate, we have a little bit of control over based on our diet history, how much food we are consuming, and then how much muscle mass we have. People who are chronic dieters typically have a slower metabolism, a lower metabolic rate, and those who have more muscle, and muscle is a tissue that requires more energy to maintain than fat, are going to burn more calories at rest. But it doesn't make as much of a difference as we often believe. Our basal metabolic rate is variable but we don't have as much control over it as many people think.

Then we have non-exercise activity thermogenesis which is where we have the most control. It's very variable from person to person. And typically, leaner individuals will just naturally move more throughout the day and it's mostly subconscious. It's more walking and fidgeting and just moving around more. We see that when in a caloric restrictive state, the NEAT levels will go down subconsciously. Our bodies are trying to protect us and one of the ways that they do that is by lowering the amount that we move throughout the day. We often see that when food and calories increase, NEAT also goes up subconsciously.

When we look at calorie balance, we try to calculate how many calories you're burning throughout the day. Of course, it's an estimate. This is not something that we can just measure and have an exact number but through tracking and figuring out maintenance, we can get a good idea of where that caloric maintenance is for each individual. There's going to be different factors like dieting history, age, activity level, gender, weight, etc that will play a role but essentially, what we want to understand is that the calories inside of the equation, is the food and drinks that we're consuming, and the calories outside of the equation is all of the calories that we're burning through those components of total daily energy expenditure.

Calories are then broken down into macronutrients. These are the only areas that calories can come from, and because we need them in large quantities, they're called macronutrients or macros. Protein has four calories per gram, carbohydrate has four calories per gram and fats have nine calories per gram. The only other place that we can get calories from outside of macros is alcohol, which has seven calories per gram. Calories are the most important driver for weight loss and weight gain. Macros are going to be important for body composition and the ratio of muscle to fat on our bodies. You can eat in a caloric deficit, lose weight, but actually not be happy with your appearance. If a lot of that weight loss is from muscle, you may be displeased with how you look. On the other hand, you can potentially stay weight stable, but end up very pleased with body composition results. If you were to gain five pounds of muscle and lose five pounds of fat, you'd obtain a leaner, more fit physique. This is why macronutrient composition is so important and the ratios of macros will depend on age, gender, training, history, goals, current body composition, personal preference and personality types. Now, protein and fats are essential nutrients meaning we need them to survive. Carbohydrates are not essential but they're certainly helpful in many different contexts like recovery, energy, and supporting thyroid and hormonal function.

So, when we look at the order of importance, first we have adherence, then we have calories, then we have macros. And next, we have micronutrients. I don't want to say that macros are more important than micronutrients because food quality is just as important as food quantity. So we're going to just say that those are equal. We often see a lot of debating over which is more important, food quantity or food quality. I would like to change the conversation and say that food quantity and food quality are equally important because they both impact each other and they both impact health and longevity. When we look at micronutrients, it's simply understanding that 50 grams of carbs coming from gummy bears will contain a very different nutrient profile than 50 grams of carbs coming from sweet potatoes. Even though you can account for calories and macros, it's important to understand the difference in food quality. Micronutrients are essential and many health issues can be solved by fixing nutrient deficiencies. A lot of people are deficient in vitamin- D, omega-3 fatty acids and magnesium, as an example.

We want to look at the foods that we're eating and understand the quality of those foods will help with any potential nutrient deficiencies. To make it simple, because micronutrients can be broken down even further into phytonutrients, flavonoids, and all these different things that are important for health, it can send you down a rabbit hole very fast. To simplify it, we just want to look at getting plenty of nutrient-rich foods in our diet, eating lots of vegetables, eating foods with a different variety of color, using different herbs and spices to flavor meals, eating different fruits and then using something to create flexibility like the 80-20 rule. This is where 80% of your food choices come from whole, nutrient-dense foods and having about 20% that are open to interpretation so you can have a little more fun with that 20%. When you're trying to be more aggressive or have a goal that requires more specificity like getting on stage for a competition, then that ratio needs to be shifted a bit. So a bodybuilder who's trying to compete, they might need to be 99% with their food choices versus the typical 80/20 and that just gives you an idea of flexibility and how it shifts based on your goals. Those are the big rocks that will always yield success and if we can nail down calorie balance while always keeping our focus on adherence and sustainability, and we can keep that growth

104

mindset in place and pay attention to food quality and food quantity. You're really going to get most of the way there.

Some of the advanced tactics that a lot of people spend time talking about are meal timing and meal frequency and also supplements. I don't want to get into those because that's like talking about adding a specific paint color on your car. The big rocks are always going to win at the end of the day. We don't want to sacrifice some of the foundational pieces just for the sake of trying to hit some of these advanced methods. Meal timing and frequency may have their place when you're trying to take things to the next level, not for the general person who just wants to be fit and healthy, understanding your metabolism, understanding calorie balance, understanding macronutrients, and understanding micronutrients will get you most of the way there.

When we look at creating that foundation for success, it all starts with mindset first, it starts with understanding adherence and sustainability because, at the end of the day, we need to perform these basics consistently over a really long period of time. We are what we repeatedly do, and creating that neurological pathway that supports our healthy habits when we consistently choose nutrient-dense foods and when we consistently choose foods that support our goals, it becomes a part of us, it becomes part of who we are. You can stop relying so much on discipline and willpower because it becomes a habit. Once the basics become a habit, that's when we can really start to see some incredible transformation.

CHAPTER 11

FOOD BUDGETING AND TRACKING

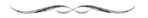

Imagine that you want to buy a new car. The first thing that you might do is look at the price and the second thing that you might do is assess what money you have coming in and what your expenses are. You want to see if you can afford that car if the budget that you're working with allows for you to take on that expense. And when we look at budgeting for something that we want, like a car or buying a gift or buying a house, we don't think twice about it. However, when it comes to our nutrition, it's often met with resistance when we talk about food budgeting. However, it can be an extremely enlightening process to take the time to track and understand your individual energy balance. And this is really the most accurate depiction that we can get using the tools at our disposal to understand your calorie needs and how to accomplish your goals. And oftentimes when we talk about tracking intake, it's met with resistance or has a negative connotation because it can be seen as too rigid or unrealistic as a lifelong endeavor. And there's definitely some validity in those arguments. For example, if you're somebody who stresses out because you don't know how to track everything to the exact gram, and it's causing you to lose sleep and you're becoming obsessive, then absolutely that is a sign that you shouldn't be tracking and it's actually a sign of disordered eating. If tracking calories feels like a chore and a major stressor, that's a sign that you really shouldn't be doing it. However, I do believe that it's a practice that everyone can benefit from by doing it at least some point once in their life, for the simple fact that it helps to gain an understanding of what your daily nutrition habits look like and it's the best form of Education for knowing what our bodies respond best to.

So understanding that when you create awareness around the foods that you're eating, you can start to connect the dots between how certain foods make you feel, or how they make you perform, or whether they give you more energy or cause you to crash. When you actually log and account for the foods that you're eating, it's much easier to connect those dots. I had a client who was recently started tracking her food and we started to talk through the process of anything that she noticed with her energy levels or her mood, or her hunger signals, and we really started to get a sense of what her body was communicating. She noticed that every day, around one o'clock she was having a major energy crash and it was the same regardless of how many hours of sleep she was getting, it was the same regardless of whether she had trained or done any exercise or not, and because she was logging her foods, we were able to look through her food logs, and see that she was eating a very high sugar, nutrient-void breakfast which was jacking up her blood sugar levels and causing a blood sugar crash which was causing her energy to tank and it made her feel like crap in the middle of the day. Now, this is something that she had been doing for a long time but never connected the dots because she had never tracked her intake. So as an educational process, it can really start to create some awareness around your nutrition habits and how foods make you feel.

It's also important as we want to understand how to read nutrition labels. A lot of people don't even know what's in the food that they're consuming. So when we track our intake, when we can actually measure what we're consuming, it starts to get us into the habit of looking at nutrition labels and seeing how many calories are in certain foods and anybody who has looked at a jar of peanut butter, and then actually weighed out one serving is probably shocked at how small one serving of peanut butter actually is. We typically take out a spoonful and we have this massive spoonful of peanut butter that could really be like 300 calories, whereas one serving is extremely small and would only be about 160 calories. So we start to realize some discrepancies in the portion sizes that we're consuming and what an actual portion size looks like. And that is another benefit to spending some time tracking is creating awareness around portion sizes. If you are measuring your food and getting an idea of how many calories are in different foods, all the sudden you can start to eyeball different things and understand what a portion size is supposed to look like and in this current food environment where portion sizes have gotten bigger and bigger and bigger without any awareness, it's very easy to understand how calorie consumption continues to climb, we continue to eat more and more food without even being aware of it because portion sizes are getting bigger. And we're in this food environment where there is an abundance of overly processed foods.

So, again, when we start to account for things, and we start to budget for our intake, it allows us to actually have more flexibility with some foods that we want to fit into our life that might not necessarily have a very rich nutrient profile. So if I wanted to have a doughnut or a cookie, understanding the caloric load that it comes with and understanding the portion size or the serving size of that cookie or donut it allows me to account for it, and it allows me to include it in my daily budget, just like I would if I was trying to budget for a new car or for a house, I would look at everything that I have coming in and what I'm spending money on. The same thing as we get to choose where we're spending that food budget. So we decide how we want to use those calories and we start to make choices based on how they serve us. So I know that for me, I like to eat in a way that allows me to feel like I had a nice big hearty meal. Well, if I'm filling my plate with very calorie-dense foods, like fast food or high sugar food, I'm not going to feel very full because the food volume is much lower. But now if I'm filling my plate with vegetables and having some fruit and lean protein and sweet potatoes, I feel like I had a nice big meal. And I have that satiety signal, I feel that fullness signal, and it's going to sustain me much longer.

So connecting the dots between how foods make you feel throughout the day and awareness around portion sizes and where you're spending that food budget, it can be a really important process to go through simply from an education standpoint.

There are studies that have looked at just how unaware we are when it comes to our nutrition habits. One study in particular showed that the participants were under-reporting their food intake by close to 50% and over-reporting their exercise by over 50%. Those are huge discrepancies in thinking that we're eating a lot less than we actually are and moving a lot more than we actually are. Creating awareness is the first step to creating change. Simply going through the process of accounting for what you're consuming can be very enlightening on many different levels.

Now, I do understand the burden that it can cause for people because having to weigh or measure your food and enter it into an app like MyFitnessPal is not exactly convenient. The way that I look at it is tracking your intake is similar to scaling Everest. When you are first starting, and you're really just focusing on some of those foundational steps, you're climbing up the mountain and you don't have to be as specific. But if we really want to get to the top of that mountain, we have to be a little bit more intentional about what we're doing. The foot placements get tougher and we have to really be more specific about what we're doing.

So I look at tracking, as we're climbing up the mountain and we've got a good way up the mountain with the basics and our habits, but now we want to spend a little bit of time becoming more specific and creating more education and awareness around what we're doing. And I think that the process of understanding your caloric needs can really help make better choices if you're somebody who doesn't want to track for a long period of time. So if maybe you just spent 30 days tracking, and you start to understand your needs, from a calorie standpoint, from a food quality standpoint, from a macronutrient standpoint. Now, all of a sudden, you're more likely to make better choices in alignment with what you're trying to accomplish when you stop tracking. So it almost helps you become more in tune with your body and connect the dots between what's going to be most sustainable for you in a way that allows for more specificity. And it's a more intentional way of doing things. It doesn't have to be a lifestyle. It doesn't have to be something that you do for a very long period of time but if you think about how long you're going to be alive, hopefully, a very long time, it's worth spending 30 days tracking intake for the amount of knowledge, education, and experience that it will provide and how that can serve your nutritional habits for the rest of your life. So it's really taking a fraction of a percent of your life and the benefit that it can create is well worth it in my opinion.

So using food tracking and budgeting, understanding how to read labels, understanding portion sizes and understanding how certain foods make you feel is a valuable thing to do for 30 days and something that I believe everybody should do at some point in their life.

CHAPTER 12

INTUITIVE EATING

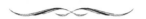

Imagine a typical morning in your day to day life where you wake up, you have to get to work, you head downstairs, you have your cup of coffee, you're trying to get the kids ready for school and you're running a little bit late, you're trying to get all of your stuff together, the kids need you, you have to pack lunches, you want to finish your coffee, you want to maybe say goodbye to your spouse. All these things are happening as you're trying to get out the door and you realize that you haven't had breakfast yet. So you rush over, you grab something from the fridge, you stand at the counter while you talk to your kids and tell them to have a great day at school, and you shove down your breakfast and head out the door.

Now, how likely in that scenario, are you to be in tune with your body's natural signals from the meal that you just ate? Do you think that you'll be very in tune with your hunger signals or feelings of satiety? Do you think that you'll be able to pay attention and appreciate the meal that you just had, and be able to mindfully eat? The likelihood is very low. And the nature of our daily lives and the amount of stress that we're under causes a challenge when it comes to eating mindfully. So we don't spend a lot of time actually sitting quietly without distractions and enjoying a meal. Hopefully, that's a practice that you still have in your daily life but for a lot of people, it's not. More and more people are eating on the run, eating in their car, standing at the counter, eating in a rush, eating while watching TV, eating while on their phones, eating while listening to a podcast. There are so many distractions that disrupt our ability to actually sit and be present and pay attention to the food that we're consuming. It makes it increasingly more challenging to intuitively eat.

Like most topics in the fitness space, intuitively eating is a heavily debated concept. A lot of people don't truly understand the ideas and framework of intuitive eating, so let's first start with a basic understanding. Although Intuitive Eating (IE) is often said to be an 'anti-diet,' this is a gross and inaccurate generalization with a myopic perspective. Intuitive Eating is a framework of self-care principles, which is designed to:

- remove the "good vs bad" labels of food

- improve your relationship with food

- remove weight stigma

- emphasize emotional & physical wellness over weight loss

- create increased awareness of hunger and satiety signals

It often goes hand-in-hand with the Health at Every Size (HAES), which promotes the concepts of:

113

- Weight inclusivity

- Health enhancement

- Respectful care

- Eating for well-being

- Life-enhancing movement

Contrary to popular belief, HAES does not state that health is present at every size. The main pillar of the movement is that a person's size should not prevent them from engaging in health-seeking behavior. They believe that weight is not predictive of health status and focus on health-seeking behaviors rather than outcomes (such as weight loss). Both HAES and IE are weight-neutral, which is not synonymous with anti-weight-loss. Any outcome, such as weight loss, weight gain, or weight stability may occur as a result of health-promoting behaviors. However, intentional weight loss is not the goal, but it may be one of the many outcomes of a lifestyle change that focuses on mental, emotional, and physical self-care. HAES establishes that informing a client or patient that they need to lose weight is just as ineffective as informing them that they need to reduce their blood pressure. Statistically speaking, both weight-loss-focused and weight-neutral programs result in very little weight loss after 6-9 months of intervention. However, both realize positive health outcomes such as improvements in cardiometabolic risk factors, and weight-neutral approaches also boast improvements in psychological health outcomes. This isn't to say that weight loss isn't beneficial. Evidence illustrates that it can be. But HOW it is achieved is arguably more important than the outcome itself, and if we can help our clients achieve better health with less physiological or psychological damage, then that is something worth exploring.

IE is often considered to be a "diet break," which is also inaccurate. Rather it is a collection of principles intended to break cycles of harmful eating behaviors and challenge the beliefs that precipitate them. It seeks to address cognitive distortions that lead to negative self-perception and chronic dieting and utilizes an evidence-based approach with an extensive body of literature in individuals with overweight, obesity, and binge eating disorder. Emerging literature is examining its use in a variety of other populations, as well, and the results are promising. IE describes the cycle of chronic dieting as phases of deprivation, rebellion, and rebound weight gain, resulting in subsequent deprivation. As someone who experienced this vicious cycle personally and successfully coached many clients out of the typical diet mentality, the integration of IE has been paramount in that success.

A diet, in this context, refers to a way of eating for the sole purpose of reducing body weight. Many individuals believe IE is simply a phase of uninhibited eating. Their reasoning is often along the lines of most individuals can't control themselves when it comes to highly palatable and highly seductive foods. Unfortunately, the combination of diet culture and misunderstanding leads people to fear and vilify the entire paradigm at the thought of weight gain and eating 'without rules or reason.' A deeper dive into the principles illustrates that any individual embarking on this journey will be doing far more internal work than most people realize or believe. The principles of IE emphasize satisfaction as the focal point during mealtimes, enjoyable physical activity, rejection of the diet mentality, using nutrition information without judgment, and respecting one's body even in the presence of negative feelings about how it might look. It is a dynamic, integrative process that appreciates the connections between our thoughts, feelings, and behaviors around nutrition and physical activity in order to facilitate positive, productive relationships with our food, physical activity, and selves.

The book "Intuitive Eating" covers ten main principles of self-care around food, physical activity, and mental well being. There are:

1. Reject the Diet Mentality

- the false hope of losing weight quickly, easily and permanently

- the lie that weight regain is failure

- the promise that there's a new or better diet that will work for you

2. Honor Your Hunger

- remain biologically fed through adequate energy intake to prevent excessive hunger that may lead to overeating and counter your intentions to eat moderately and consciously

- learn to respond to biological hunger to rebuild your trust in self around food

- eating when hungry, rather than in response to a specific set of rules

3. Make Peace with Food

- unconditional permission to eat in prevents feelings of deprivation and subsequent bingeing (also known as the abstinence violation effect)

- habituation through regular exposure dilutes the alluring quality of forbidden foods whereas rigid rules trigger rebellion

- eating without obligatory penance

4. Challenge the Food Police

- reject the idea of "good or bad" foods (also known as binary thinking) and food morality to reduce guilt after eating

- ignore inappropriate comments from others and liberate yourself from justifying food choices to others (or yourself)

5. Feel Your Fullness

- listen for signals that tell you you're no longer hungry

- pause mid-meal to reassess your enjoyment and fullness

- practice conscious (mindful) eating

6. Discover the Satisfaction Factor

- Eat what you really want, in an inviting environment, and focus on the pleasure of the meal in concert with your biological cues

- Savor your meal so you aren't left seeking other foods to 'hit the spot'

7. Cope with Your Emotions Without Using Food

- truly assess and meet your emotional and mental needs without food

- food can't fulfill emotional or mental needs; applying it this way may only add the discomfort of overeating to those difficult emotions and you'll have to deal with the discomfort of the overeating and those emotions

8. Respect Your Body

- recognize and accept your genetic blueprint and predispositions

- it is difficult to reject the diet mentality if you are overly critical of your body shape and unrealistic about your expectations

- respecting your body means taking care of your health, treating it with dignity and meeting its basic needs

9. Exercise (Feel the Difference)

- replace militant exercise with enjoyable physical activity

- focus on the benefits of movement rather than the calorie burn

- focusing on your enjoyment of the opportunity to move—rather than an external motivator like weight loss—will be a stronger motivator in the moment

10. Honor Your Health with Gentle Nutrition

- make food choices that honor your health, taste buds, and digestive comfort so they feel good

- you don't have to eat a "perfect" diet to be healthy; no single food is inherently going to make or break a healthy lifestyle

- emphasize moderation, balance, and a variety of fruits and vegetables, nutrient-dense foods, protein-rich foods, quality fats, and whole foods; processed foods are generally less nutrient-dense

- balance is something to be achieved over a period of time, and it does not have to be reached at each meal; focus on consistency and progress

- at times it is appropriate to prioritize the nutritional qualities of foods *and* eat intuitively

The book also characterizes potential types of 'dieters' based on common beliefs and habits. The Careful Eater is militant and diligent, enforcing strict rules that, when broken, lead to bingeing behaviors. The Professional Eater may have more content knowledge than the Careful Eater, but applies it for the purposes of weight loss, and may rapidly shift from one diet to the next. An Unconscious Eater is a multitasker, eating without awareness of hunger or satiety cues, often cleaning the plate or perhaps eating emotionally. The Intuitive Eater eats in response to biological cues, making choices without guilt and enjoys the pleasure of eating while respecting their fullness.

Understandably, the transition from cyclic, chronic dieting to a normal eating pattern that responds to physiological hunger without the structure of specific dietary guidelines is daunting for many. The book outlines some common experiences which likely resonate with many individuals. Importantly, the "Exploration" phase seems to create the most confusion and controversy, as it's often the only one that people imagine experiencing. However, this clarifies that the commonly-held belief, "I can eat whatever I want, as much as I want, whenever I feel like it," distorts the premise of IE because this can lead to physical discomfort and is not satisfying. The stages, while not necessarily linear, do lend themselves to a processional flow as one might reach complete diet burnout before embarking upon IE.

1. Hitting Diet Bottom:

- feelings of failure, frustration, discouragement, and being "stuck"

- negative body image

- unintentional weight gain

- lost touch with physical cues of hunger and fullness (interoceptive awareness)

- strict food rules and emotion dictate food choices

- weary of dieting but terrified of eating

- cycles of restriction and counterregulatory eating (the "Last Supper" phenomenon leads to excessive intake of 'off-limits' food due to perceived past and future restriction)

2. Exploration

- conscious learning and pursuit of pleasure

- Hyper consciousness and awareness of mind and body cues

- experimentation with new foods; with permission comes choice

- reconnecting with physical cues

- It may be difficult to respect fullness due to old thoughts of deprivation and difficulty recognizing the appropriate level of fullness

- not indicative of lifetime habits, but a period of time learning

3. Crystallization

- feeling like solid behavior change

- thoughts are no longer obsessive

- easier to identify and respond to physical cues

- more established trust in self

4. The Intuitive Eater Awakens

- comfortable and free-flowing

- consistently and easily choose what you want when biologically hungry and stopping when full, so food is more satisfying

- healthier foods are chosen because they feel better rather than any moral value

- you have found alternative outlets for emotions, so they no longer dictate your food choices

5. Treasure the Pleasure

- feeling empowered, regularly practicing positive self-talk and trust

- nutrition and exercise are paths to health and feeling good

- this lifestyle is enjoyable and enticing

The benefits of IE and other HAES-aligned weight-neutral approaches to health are documented in literature, and span both physical and psychological outcomes. While weight-focused programs do result in greater weight loss at 6 or 9-month follow-ups, long-term studies illustrate higher attrition rates in dieting groups and little or no significant difference in net weight loss. A recent meta-analysis reported that, after 4-5 years, individuals in structured weight-loss programs maintained a 3.2% reduction in body weight, which was only slightly more than those on the weight-neutral program. It's very apparent that unsustainable diets produce unsustainable results, and with such a heightened emphasis on weight loss as an outcome, the process of getting there is often overlooked. More importantly, dieting behaviors predict later development of disordered eating — a phenomenon that isn't currently identified in weight-neutral approaches.

One question that challenges practitioners, that you may be wondering as well, is the question of metabolically healthy obesity (MHO). Is it factual? A recent meta-analysis found that the prevalence of metabolically healthy obesity is about 35% in individuals with obesity, though they do have an 80% increased relative risk of developing a metabolic abnormality within 3-10 years, and about half of them will no longer be considered metabolically healthy over time. The facts about metabolic disease risk factors can be used to inform, but shouldn't be used to stigmatize. We must acknowledge that MHO is as real as weight stigma, and approach the conversation conscientiously.

What about the physical outcomes of weight-neutral approaches?

Weight-neutral (WN) approaches such as eating in response to biological hunger and the use of fasting blood glucose measurement has been shown to improve insulin sensitivity and lead to weight loss in individuals receiving diabetes education. Contrary to popular belief, high scores on the Intuitive Eating Scale don't correlate with an increase in unhealthy food or BMI; in fact, a study on members of the US Army illustrated correlations between normal BMI, intuitive eating scores, and eating in response to biological hunger. The phenomenon of greater reliance on hunger signals is consistent across the literature in individuals with overweight and obesity, as well. This is an intriguing finding in light of the fact that some studies have illustrated that individuals dealing with being overweight, obesity, or anorexia nervosa exhibit attenuated hunger and satiety signals, resulting in a level of food intake that may not match energy needs. When comparing cardiometabolic markers such as blood lipids and blood pressure, long-term studies illustrate no differences in improvements between weight-neutral and weight-loss programs. Compared to weight-loss approaches, weight-neutral approaches significantly reduce episodes of binge eating and bulimia scores. This could be due, in part, to the habituation response to repeated food exposure which leads to reduced food novelty, making it less tempting. In concert with mindful eating, this can reduce distracted, counterregulatory eating which may lead to eating past fullness, which is commonly seen during chronic dieting cycles. Importantly, because weight-neutral approaches focus on behaviors, individuals participating in these programs increase their physical activity levels and dietary quality.

Healthy habits such as consuming fruits and vegetables, exercising, limiting alcohol intake, and refraining from smoking can improve health independent of BMI. In fact, low cardiorespiratory fitness is a stronger predictor of all-cause mortality risk than BMI.

What about the mental outcomes of weight-neutral approaches?

Participation in weight-neutral programs significantly reduces body dissatisfaction, dieting attempts, eating disorder symptoms, and depressive symptoms. Multiple studies in males and females have found associations between IE scores and positive body image, unconditional self-regard, and a focus on body function rather than appearance, among many other beneficial psychological variables. While these are correlational in nature and not all studies can discern directionality between IE and psychological outcomes, longitudinal studies have identified IE as a predictor for reduced risk of developing low self-esteem and engaging in unhealthy weight-loss behaviors. Interestingly, positive self-talk and encouragement (specifically after weight regain) was recently identified as a key behavior in individuals successfully maintaining weight long-term. In contrast, restrained eating can precipitate binge/purge cycles and increase the risk of developing an eating disorder. Given the risk of developing disordered eating as a result of engaging in diet behaviors and the elevated prevalence of eating disorders in the athletic population, these results should not be overlooked.

A skill-set within the framework of, but not exclusive to, IE is that of mindful eating. Mindful eating can be described as "eating with *attention* and *intention*." The Center for Mindful Eating provides the following principles:

- becoming aware of positive and nurturing opportunities available through food preparation and consumption

- respecting one's inner wisdom around food selection

- choosing to eat food that is nourishing and pleasing

- using all senses to explore food

- awareness and use of physical hunger and satiety signals to guide the beginning and end of a meal

Mindfulness is commonly perceived as a trait someone might possess, but it is more likely a skill that arises as both a function of an individual's capacity for self-regulation and their motivation to enact that self-regulation. Motivation to allocate these mental resources depends on an individual's belief in the value of mindfulness *and* their ability to allocate mental resources to remaining mindful. Mindfulness requires attention, reflection, and practice. It is arguably one of the more valuable but overlooked skills we can encourage clients or patients to practice. By establishing a strong inner framework and intentionality behind our actions, we can make choices aligned with our goals and values regardless of the external environment. This is why we developed the Nutritional Mindfulness course, which provides our clients with the opportunity to actively take part in the practice of mindful eating.

We encourage our students to ask themselves probing questions about why they want to eat, when they want to eat, how they usually eat, what they eat, how much they eat, and where they invest their energy from eating. While these seem simple on the surface, we are actually asking students to think about whether or not they're eating for biological hunger, how often they're thinking about food, how mindfully they're consuming their food, what dictates their food choices and intake, and whether their current relationship with food might be overruling their ability to be fully present in their lives.

Similar to the phases covered in Intuitive Eating, Michelle May, M.D. describes specific types of eaters: Instinctive, Overeating, and Restrictive. Instinctive eaters fuel their bodies in response to biological hunger with an awareness of nutrition but no emotional attachment to the food and they consume meals with intentionality, purpose, and focus so they can direct their energy to live an active life. Overeaters and Restrictive eaters may eat based on rules, triggers, or emotions, and their meals may be consumed mindlessly, rigidly, or even in secret. Unlike Instinctive eaters, they often find themselves reinvesting their energy back into the dieting cycle, or simply storing the excess fuel that isn't used.

Mindful eating cultivates non-judgment and self-acceptance, and though this is aimed at mealtimes, it can be applied to all facets of life. While it may lead to weight loss, the focus is still placed on other health-based   outcomes.

There still appears to be a sea of doubt over individuals' abilities to

128

apply interoceptive awareness at mealtimes. The doubt and criticism surrounding IE and HAES likely also stem from a misunderstanding, lack of awareness, and perhaps some fear. Intuitive eating is not synonymous with eating without rational thought, or eating based on emotion or eating as much as one possibly can of everything they might want (though all of these things might happen...but they might happen regardless). Applying the principles of intuitive eating facilitates the disruption of harmful eating patterns and cycles. Intuitive eating is not a diet. It's a foundation of principles creating a collective approach to modify behavior for a more beneficial outcome. Obviously, IE is about much more than eating, but it is in this arena that we can begin to build a shared understanding and improve the dialogue around all aspects of IE and HAES.

We might start by considering that biological cues *can* regulate food intake and that everyone would benefit by not *needing* to rationalize a food choice based on external influence.

We might also be able to agree that mindful eating is a skillset, and a form of autoregulation in eating.

Perhaps we can also agree that awareness, adaptation, and flexibility in our approach to eating, training, and coaching ultimately lead to better outcomes.

Most of all, I hope we can agree that our vigilant focus on the external environment and factors that drive behavior has led to neglecting the internal environment—the one that is truly within our capacity to change and fortify. By investing in the internal environments, our clients and we can more effectively respond to the external when it's out of our control.

We have already seen a paradigm shift away from rigid attempts to control long-term outcomes, instead of remaining flexible and in charge of the current situation in order to remain on a generally positive trajectory.

Many people believe that they have to be on one side of the spectrum or the other. In other words, they believe that you have to choose between tracking food intake and macros for the rest of your life or fully practicing intuitive eating. I believe both have their place in the proper context, depending on the individual. As with most things nutrition-related, we are led to believe it's an "either-or" decision, when in reality it can be both. Self-love and wanting to change aren't mutually exclusive. Some individuals can benefit greatly from tracking their food and their workouts. Some individuals can benefit greatly from backing away from tracking and moving to an intuitive approach. It is possible to hang out in both camps or move seamlessly between them. It's not about one being "right" and the other being "wrong." It's about what's right for you, at this current stage of your life. That can and likely will change over time.

In fact, food budgeting and macro tracking can be a great entry point into intuitive eating again, because now we've created awareness around portion sizes, we've created awareness around how certain foods make us feel. And we've created the awareness around hyper-palatable foods and the impact they have on us. So now we can manage portion size, and we can start to eat intuitively again, by having that education and understanding. Now we can take the time to really practice and learn intuitive eating based on our current lifestyle. So if we look at tracking calories and macros like climbing to the top of Everest, intuitive eating is like coming down from that summit and getting to the other side safely and effectively and having that accomplishment last forever. So we've achieved this pinnacle of success. And now we want to sustain it. But we want to do it in a way that doesn't cause additional stress. Therefore, tracking might not be a lifelong endeavor. So we can implement and practice mindful eating to sustain our forever solution. It's an important practice to go through, as it will actually improve your quality of life. It will improve your relationships, it will improve your ability to connect with people and it will allow you to be much more in tune with what your body wants and needs. And we understand that it's an individual process. It's really the internal work that is going to set you on the path to success and to ultimately achieve diet freedom.

In conclusion, we know that diets don't work. I should say that diets don't work the way that they're traditionally set up. We have firm statistics on that, where only 5% of people who go through a diet protocol will actually sustain the weight that they lost for more than three years. However, just saying that diets don't work might foster the idea that you shouldn't even bother to make a change, which is the opposite of the mindset that we want to encourage. Remember that we're building a growth mindset. So you already know that your belief in yourself is going to go a long way into creating change, but we want to create change the right way. Therefore, avoiding the typical fad diets and removing the all or nothing mindset, or having a start date and an end date are all important steps to take. We want to approach this process from a behavior change standpoint that is sustainable and that's going to last you a lifetime with the understanding that one size does not fit all.

Our personality type tells us a lot about what will and what won't work so we can use that information to create a protocol that makes you feel your best, perform your best, look your best, and achieve the level of health that you want to accomplish. We may have to do some experimentation, we may have to continue to tweak the process to find that sweet spot for you, but the end result is well worth it. The end result means that you never have to diet again. The end result is that you never have to worry about any more failed dieting attempts. The end result is that you don't have to fall for quick fixes that you see everybody else around you doing, knowing that they're going to rebound in a short period after the diet is over. And the ultimate place that you land is in a place of better health and becoming the best version of you.

So welcome home, you have now found your forever solution. And I invite you to visit the website to take these results to the next level and put them into action.

THANK YOU FOR READING MY BOOK!

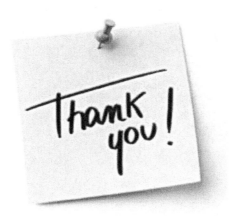

FREE BONUS GIFT

Just to say thanks for buying and reading my book, I would like to give you a free bonus gift that will add value and that you will appreciate, 100% FREE, no strings attached!

To Download Now, Visit:

http://www.personalitydietbook.com/MM/freegift

I appreciate your interest in my book and I value your feedback as it helps me improve future versions of this book. I would appreciate it if you could leave your invaluable review on Amazon.com with your feedback. Thank you!

Made in the USA
Middletown, DE
06 May 2020

93849322R00080